I0415830

Plan and Operation of the HANES I Augmentation Survey of Adults 25-74 Years

United States, 1974-1975

DHEW Publication No. (PHS) 78-1314

U.S. DEPARTMENT OF HEALTH, EDUCATION, AND WELFARE
Public Health Service
National Center for Health Statistics
Hyattsville, Md.   June 1978

NATIONAL CENTER FOR HEALTH STATISTICS

DOROTHY P. RICE, Director

ROBERT A. ISRAEL, Deputy Director
JACOB J. FELDMAN, Ph.D., Associate Director for *Analysis*
GAIL F. FISHER, Ph.D., *Associate* Director for the Cooperative *Health Statistics* System
ELIJAH L. WHITE, *Associate Director for Data Systems*
JAMES T. BAIRD, JR., Ph.D., *Associate Director for International Statistics*
ROBERT C. HUBER, *Associate Director for Management*
MONROE G. SIRKEN, Ph.D., *Associate Director for Mathematical Statistics*
PETER L. HURLEY, *Associate Director for Operations*
JAMES M. ROBEY, Ph.D., *Associate Director for Program Development*
PAUL E. LEAVERTON, Ph.D., *Associate Director for Research*
ALICE HAYWOOD, *Information Officer*

DIVISION OF HEALTH EXAMINATION STATISTICS

MICHAEL A. W. HATTWICK, M.D., *Director*
JEAN ROBERTS, *Chief, Medical Statistics Branch*
SIDNEY ABRAHAM, *Chief, Nutritional Statistics Branch*
LINCOLN OLIVER, *Chief, Psychological Statistics Branch*
ROBERT S. MURPHY, *Chief, Survey Planning and Development Branch*

Under the legislation establishing the National Health Survey, the Public Health Service is authorized to use, insofar as possible, the services or facilities of other Federal, State, or private agencies. In accordance with specifications established by the National Center for Health Statistics, the U.S. Bureau of the Census participated in the design and selection of the sample and carried out the household interview stage of the data collection and certain parts of the statistical processing.

The Center for Disease Control acted as laboratory consultants and performed a series of biochemical, hematological, and serological assessments on blood **specimens** of persons participating in the survey.

The U.S. Environmental Protection Agency supervised the chemical analyses of the water samples collected at each household.

Vital and Health Statistics-Series I-No. 14

DHEW Publication No. (PHS) 78-1314
Library of Congress Catalog Card Number 78-606016

ACKNOWLEDGMENTS

Special acknowledgment is due Mr. Arthur J. McDowell, former Director of the Division of Health Examination Statistics, and Dr. Jean-Pierre Habicht, former Special Assistant to the Director, for their guidance in the formulation of the HANES I Augmentation Survey.

CONTENTS

LIST OF FIGURES

SYMBOLS

Data not available-- - - -

Category not applicable------------------------------- . . .

Quantity zero-- -

Quantity more than 0 but less than 0.05------ 0.0

Figure does not meet standards of
   reliability or precision------------------------------- *

PLAN AND OPERATION OF THE HANES I AUGMENTATION SURVEY OF ADULTS 25-74 YEARS

Arnold Engel, M.D., Robert S. Murphy, Kurt Maurer, and Everette Collins,
Division of Health Examination Statistics

INTRODUCTION

In the Health Examination Survey (HES), a major program of the National Center for Health Statistics (NCHS), data are collected by direct physical examination, tests, and measurements performed on the sample population studied. The National Health Survey was authorized under the National Health Survey Act of 1956 by the 84th Congress to be a continuous public health service activity to monitor the health status of the American population. Information has been obtained on the prevalence of certain medically defined illnesses and the distribution of a variety of physical, physiological, and psychological measurements. The Survey provides this information for the U.S. civilian noninstitutionalized population and simultaneously provides the demographic and socioeconomic data necessary for analysis. In recent years, procedures to measure either directly or indirectly the impact of the environment on individuals and to delineate met and unmet health care needs have been employed in the Survey.

The first three national surveys conducted between 1959 and 1970 had specific age groupings as their target populations. These were adults ages 18-79 years, children ages 6-11, and youths ages 12-17.[1-3] The fourth survey program, the first Health and Nutrition Examination Survey (HANES I) was conducted between April 1971 and June 1974 on a probability sample of the U.S. noninstitutionalized civilian population, ages 1-74. An extensive nutrition examination and special examinations by ophthalmologists, dermatologists, and dentists were given to every sample person who was examined. Additional examination components focused on other aspects of health were administered to a subsample of adults (25-74 years), about one-fifth of all the examinees. These additional components were designated as the "detailed" components, in contrast with the somewhat simpler nutrition examinations.

A reduction in the magnitude of resources available for conducting the field operation made it necessary to cut back the number of field teams from three to two in January 1973. It had originally been anticipated that the detailed components would be continued into a second HANES program. Due to the reduction in field teams, HANES I required 3 years instead of 2. In order to speed up the availability of the data from detailed components, it was decided to devote the 15-month period, July 1974 through September 1975, to approximately double the number of people examined for the detailed health component. The larger sample size would facilitate analysis of the examination findings by smaller demographic groupings. In addition, the prolonged period of data collection would also provide more time for planning the design of the next projected Health and Nutrition Examination Survey (HANES II) so as to take greater advantage of information and experience gained from HANES I. This 15-month operation was referred to as the "Augmentation Survey" for the detailed component.

For the 15-month augmentation phase of the detailed component of HANES I, a number of changes were made in both the content of the examination and the sample design. The operation of the survey proceeded in roughly the same manner as it did in the first part of HANES I. The purpose of this report is to supplement the program description of HANES I[4] by describing the modifications in procedures, program content, sampling, and other data collection activities that were made for the augmentation phase of HANES I. Stand sequencing, scheduling, professional and public relations, logistical arrangements, household interviewing, appointment procedures, quality control, examination procedures, and the composition of the field staff are described in the HANES I program report. Most of the components of the detailed examination were continued with little or no modification. For a detailed discussion of the components in the following listing, reference to the HANES I program description[4] is advised. A description of the nutrition and special examinations given in HANES I and copies of the forms used in HANES I are also included. Copies of the forms used in the HANES I Augmentation Survey are found in appendix III of this report. Detailed instructions and procedures used in HANES I and the HANES I Augmentation Survey are described in the staff instruction manuals, which are available upon request.[5-7]

Components of the HANES I Detailed Examination Survey that were continued in the HANES I Augmentation Survey include:

1. A physician's examination.

2. Spirometry.

3. Single-breath carbon monoxide test for pulmonary diffusion.

4. A 12-lead electrocardiogram (ECG).

5. Pure-tone audiometry at 500, 1,000, 2,000, and 4,000 cycles.

6. Anthropometric measurements.

7. Medical History, General Medical History Supplement, Health Care Needs, Arthritis, Respiratory, and Cardiovascular questionnaires.

8. A schedule for measuring psychological well-being.

9. Hand-wrist X-rays processed for bone density and cortical thickness and hip and knee X-rays assessed for the presence of arthritis.

10. Laboratory tests--Serum: Measurements of SCOT, alkaline phosphatase, bilirubin, uric acid, folates, cholesterol, calcium, phosphorus, and serology tests for measles, German measles, polio, tetanus, diphtheria, and amebiasis were performed. Whole *blood:* Hematocrit, hemoglobin, red and white cell counts, and white cell differential count were continued. Hemoglobinopathy screening that was instituted during the conduct of HANES I was also continued in the Augmentation Survey.

NEW PROCEDURES

Hearing Test for Speech

The purpose of this test was to provide a measure of the ability of the U.S. population to hear and understand conversational speech.

Recommendations for the addition of the test came from a number of speech and hearing authorities who attended an advisory meeting at NCHS. These included Hallowell Davis, Central Institute for the Deaf; Leo Doeffler, Stanley Zerling, and Ralph Nauton, University of Chicago; and Eldon Eagles, Associate Director for the National Institute of Neurological and Communicative Disorders and Stroke, National Institutes of Health.

The stimuli used in the test consisted of the revised Central Institute for the Deaf Sentences supplied by Dr. Davis. The material was developed by a working group of the Committee on Hearing and Bioacoustics of the National Research Council. The following criteria were followed in developing 10 lists of 10 sentences each:

Vocabulary appropriate to adults.

Words that appear with high frequency as cited in one or more of the well-known word counts of the English language.

Exclusion of proper names and proper nouns.

Free use of common nonslang idioms and constructions.

Avoidance of phonetic loading and tongue twisting.

High redundancy.

Low level of abstraction.

Grammatical construction that varies freely.

The sentences in each list contained 50 keywords (appendix III, forms Q and R). The keywords are shown in capital letters in each of the sentences. The recordings of the sentences made under contract at the University of Maryland by Dr. G. Donald Causey were examined at the National Bureau of Standards and judged to be of excellent technical quality.

In the test format, the initial list of sentences was presented at a level 10-15 decibels (dB) below the 100-cycle pure-tone threshold unless that threshold was 25 dB or lower. In that case, testing always began at the 20-dB level. Depending on the results of the initial presentation, the next list was presented at either 10 dB higher or 10 dB lower. The end-point for terminating the test was the correct identification of 90 percent of the keywords in a particular list. A different list was presented at each 10-dB level within the range of 20 dB to 80 dB, as determined by the degree of hearing loss.

Vision Testing

The inclusion of visual acuity tests in the HANES I Augmentation Survey was for the purpose of comparing objective tests of visual disability with a series of questions designed for the same purpose. The near-vision test used in the examination was designed to measure one's ability to read printed selections. Keeney and Sloan cards had different style typefaces and different reading selections. Using both Keeney and Sloan cards together provided a wide range of type sizes for testing near-vision acuity. An adaptation of the test provided some information on near vision for illiterate persons.

Distance visual acuity was measured in previous examination programs by using devices that simulated the recommended 20-foot distance—by optical methods such as the use of mirrors. Since some inaccuracies are introduced by the use of distance simulation devices, it was decided to use Good-lite charts at an actual 20-foot distance. Carefully controlled direct and background lighting was used to ensure accuracy. Both binocular and monocular distance vision were tested.

Water Sample Collaborative Study (HANES-National Institutes of Health-Environmental Protection Agency)

This study was undertaken to evaluate the possible relationships among bulk constituents, hardness, and trace metals in household tapwater with certain risk factors of cardiovascular disease. Water samples were collected from taps or wells and from public water distribution supplies. The samples are being analyzed by the Environmental Protection Agency to measure their hardness, alkalinity, and the total amount of solute present. They are also being tested for the presence and concentration of sizable numbers of trace minerals. In addition to the water sample collection, a questionnaire (appendix III, form C) was administered to the sample persons detailing personal consumption of water and the source of the water supplied to the household. The water pipes under the sink were examined to determine their composition.

Additional Questionnaire Material

During the Health Interview Survey (HIS), conducted annually by NCHS, approximately 40,000 households are interviewed to obtain a wide variety of health information. Sets of questions on vision and hearing developed for HIS were included in the HANES exam. This would enable HIS to provide a better basis for interpretation of the relationship of a person's answers to questionnaires in these fields to clinical findings. In short, the questionnaire items provide a scaled index of impairment for hearing, distance visual acuity, and reading ability (appendix III, form B).

A portion of the 1975 HIS schedule on hypertension was included so that it could be correlated with the clinical data obtained in the HANES I Augmentation Survey. A final addition was a 20-question depression scale that the National Institute of Mental Health recommended to be included. This scale had been used in two large community studies. Since depression is an exceedingly common and important condition for study, the epidemiological relationship of it to various other health factors is of considerable interest.

Additional Laboratory Procedures

Because of continuous interest in monitoring the prevalence of venereal disease in the U.S. population, serological tests for syphilis were added to the survey. These tests, performed at the Center for Disease Control consisted of the ART, VDRL, and FTA. Another study subject was hemoglobinopathies. Tests for hemoglobinopathies were actually begun on a special pilot basis at the 37th location of HANES I. Although considerable information is available from local studies, interest was shown in developing estimates for the U.S. population. The laboratory procedure performed involved the phenotyping of red cells. On the SMA 12/60, the additional determinations of blood urea nitrogen (BUN), creatinine, sodium, and potassium were done. The BUN and serum creatinine levels served as indicators of kidney impairment in the population.

SAMPLE DESIGN

The sample design for the HANES I Augmentation Survey of Adults had two basic requirements: The sample of persons selected for examination in locations 66-100 would constitute a national probability sample of the target population and, when considered jointly with those receiving the detailed examination in HANES I locations 1-65, the sample would be a 100-PSU (primary sampling unit), national probability sample. All 100 of the HANES sample locations are listed in appendix II by geographic region and probability design. As indicated in appendix II, 10 of the PSU's were included in both the Augmentation Survey sample and in the initial 65-PSU design, so that actually there were only 90 distinct sample PSU's. The sample design specifications, selection procedures, and

data collection procedures for the first 65 PSU's are described elsewhere.[4] Definitions relating to the sample design and selection of locations remained constant throughout the 100 survey locations.

The HANES I Augmentation Survey sample was designed to meet the following goals:

1. To examine a national probability sample of adults 25-74 years of age which represents the civilian noninstitutionalized population of the contiguous United States, excluding those living on lands set aside for use by American Indians.

2. To complete the survey of approximately 4,300 sample persons in a 12- to 15-month period.

3. To sample the target population in proportion to its representation in the population-with no oversampling of special groups.

4. To produce two kinds of estimates from the survey: (a) distributions of the population by specified characteristics such as blood pressure and selected biochemical determinations; and (b) prevalence in the population of selected chronic conditions, particularly arthritic, respiratory, and cardiovascular conditions.

5. To set maximum tolerances for variability for these key statistics permitting a general analysis by broad geographic regions and by other major demographic subgroups such as income, race, age, and sex.

Selection of Primary Sampling Units

The program description of HANES I[4] describes the contiguous United States as divided into 1,900 geographic areas or PSU's. These 1,900 PSU's were collapsed into 357 strata for HIS and collapsed again into 40 superstrata for HANES. Of these 40 superstrata, 15 are composed of only 1 very large metropolitan area of more than 2 million people and were drawn into the HANES 65-PSU design with certainty. However, in the Augmentation Survey only five of them were drawn into the sample with certainty :

Essex, Morris, Union, Somerset, Hudson, Middlesex, N. J.

Essex, Middlesex, Norfolk, Plymouth, Suffolk, Mass.

Allegheny, Beaver, Washington, Westmoreland, Pa.

Macomb, Oakland, Wayne, Mich.

Alameda, Contra-Costa, San Mateo, San Francisco, Solano, Calif.

The other 10 superstrata that were drawn into the 65-PSU design with certainty were collapsed into 5 groups of two each, only 1 of which was chosen for the Augmentation Survey with a probability of 0.5:

Nassau, Queens, Suffolk, N.Y.

Bronx, N.Y.

Bucks, Chester, Delaware, Montgomery, Philadelphia, Pa.

Lake, Porter, Cook, Will, Kane, Ill.

Orange, Los Angeles, Calif.

However, when these five locations are considered as part of the 100-PSU design they are selected with certainty.

In each of the 25 remaining noncertainty strata, defined as they were for the HANES I 65-PSU design," a selection of a PSU was made with probability proportional to size in a controlled selection procedure, independent of its selection status in the 65-PSU design. Only two PSU's in the noncertainty strata were included in both surveys:

St. Bernard, Jefferson, Orleans, La.

Hancock, Hamblen, Hawkins, Claiborne, Tenn.

Sample Selection Within Primary Sampling Units

Within PSU's, using 1970 census data, enumeration districts (ED's) were divided into segments of an expected eight housing units each.

In urban areas where listing units were well defined in 1970, this division was quite accurate, since the sampling frame was comprised of listings that resulted from the 1970 census. For ED's not covered by the listing books, area sampling was employed, and consequently, some variation in segment size occurred. To make the sample representative of the current population of the United States, the listed segments were supplemented by a sample of housing units that had been constructed since 1970. Then a systematic sample of segments in each PSU was selected. Randomly selected reserve segments were drawn to provide a minimum of 105 sample persons per PSU.

After the sample segments had been identified, a list of all current addresses within the segment boundaries was made, and the household interviews were conducted to determine the age of each household member, as well as to obtain other demographic and socioeconomic information required for the survey. After listing the household members according to specified rules of relationship to the head of the household, those 25-74 years of age were then added to the appropriate Sample Person Selection Sheet (figure 1) from which one of every two eligible persons was selected for participation in the survey. The sheet illustrates one of two possible sampling patterns with selection of the first listed person in the segment, third, and so forth. The patterns were randomly assigned to segments in order to effectively remove sampling bias from the selection process. The census interviewer proceeded to arrange an examination appointment for all sample persons who indicated a willingness to be examined.

Logistical arrangements, household interviewing procedures, appointment and transportation procedures, and general mobile examination center procedures are described elsewhere.4

DATA COLLECTION

Census interviewers replaced Health Examination Representatives in administering most of the material in the medical history forms as a part of the initial household interview phase of the survey. Because of this change in interviewers, the task of asking certain "sensitive" questions (e.g., those relating to kidney and

U.S. DEPARTMENT OF COMMERCE
BUREAU OF THE CENSUS

a. HES Stand Name

b. HES Stand Number

. SAMPLE PERSON SELECTION SHEET
HEALTH EXAMINATION SURVEY

c. Interviewer's Name

Part I – SAMPLE PERSON SELECTION

Line No. (1)	HH EP's Line No. (2)	Serial No. (3)	Segment No. (4)	Line No. (1)	HH EP's Line No. (2)	Serial No. (3)	Segment No. (4)	Line No. (1)	HH EP's Line No, (2)	Serial No. (3)	Segment No. (4)
①				⑮				㉙			
2				16				30			
③				⑰				㉛			
4				18				32			
⑤				⑲				㉝			
6				20				34			
⑦				㉑				㉟			
8				22				36			
⑨				㉓				㊲			
10				24				38			
⑪				㉕				㊳			
12				26				40			
⑬				㉗				㊶			
14				28				42			

Part II – CALL BACK HOUSEHOLDS *(Cross off when household is interviewed)*

Segment No. (1)	Serial No. (2)	EP's (Est.) (3)	Segment No. (1)	Serial No. (2)	EP's (Est.) (3)	Segment No. (1)	Serial No. (2)	E P's (Est.) (3)	Remarks

Figure 1. Sample Person Selection Sheet

bowel function) was given to the examining physician. There were also small modifications in the mobile units, such as the installation of 'special lighting and recording equipment. In place of scheduling 10 examinees (2 for the detailed and 8 for the nutrition exams scheduled for each of the 2 daily sessions of HANES I), 6 examinees, all for the detailed, were scheduled for each session. The average number of examinees scheduled at each location in the Augmentation Survey was 120. The lengths of time spent in different locations were roughly equal, in contrast to HANES I in which some locations had a much larger sample size than others and so required a longer stay. Because of the dropping of the dental, dermatological, and ophthalmological exams, none of the personnel responsible for these parts of the exam was present in the detailed Augmentation Survey. Nutritionists were also not needed, since the Augmentation Survey did not include a dietary history.

Quality control measures were in general similar to those outlined in *Plan and Operation of the Health and Nutrition Examination Survey*, Series 1, No. 10a.[4] Some additional procedures had been worked out during HANES I and were applied in the detailed exam for the Augmentation Survey sample as follows:

1. *X-ray technique:* Chest X-ray films were reviewed by a supervisory technician who furnished a checklist of particular errors of technique (figure 2). These were used for further instruction of the technicians. The hip and knee X-rays were graded for quality by one of the expert readers at the same time the film was being examined for pathology. In addition, listings of errors in technique in hip and knee films and in the hand-wrist X-ray films were also provided by the respective contractors on a regular

POSTERIOR-ANTERIOR CHEST FILM																
Stand ____ / Sample number	Date	Tech number	Apices not shown or cut off	Costophrenic angles not shown or cut off	Rotation of examinee	Exposure not on full inspir. (no 10 ribs)	Underexposed	Overexposed	Movement or breathing	Artifacts	Marker not shown or number incorrect	2 films taken	3 films taken	WORKSHEET A For Chief Health Technician COMMENTS	Technician signature
1															
2															
3															
4															
5															
6															
7															
8															
9															
10															
11															
12															
13															
14															
15															
16															
17															
18															

Figure 2. Quality control review form

basis. Field evaluations of the X-ray units included checking the horizontal accuracy of the X-ray beams at the beginning of a stand and using metal wedges and bone phantoms for checking the calibration of the X-ray machines for the hand and wrist bone density determinations.

2. *Spirometry:* The spirometry output was monitored on an oscilloscope. Based on morphology and reproducibility of the forced expiration trials, various corrective actions were undertaken by the technician. About 4 months after the continuation exams began, the acquisition of two-channel Gould Records provided the means of ensuring a more accurate check on the quality of the recordings.

3. *Carbon monoxide (CO) diffusion test:* The tracings from the test were reviewed to determine whether the trials were acceptable. The trials were reviewed for such items as inspiration time, breath-holding time, inspired volume/vital capacity ratio, minimum dead space washout, minimum volume of gas collected, presence of inhalation artifacts.

4. *ECG tracings:* These tracings were checked for "noise," correct lead placement, machine problems, calibration standards, and baseline shift in the field, and also on a spot basis at headquarters.

5. *Body measurements:* Body measurements were replicated as in the first 65 locations of HANES I. In addition, a random assignment of examinees to technicians within a field team was coupled with computer monitoring to compare results among technicians for body measurements.

6. *Audiometry:* The random assignment of examinees to technicians and the monitoring of technician differences were also used to compare pure-tone audiometry results. In addition, the results of the speech test were reviewed at headquarters for each stand on a regular basis and compared with the results of the pure-tone audiometry.

7. *Leg length measurements:* This X-ray determination was part of the arthritis exam. In order to ensure the accuracy of leg length determinations by X-ray, a metal stand on which the examinee stood was verified as level every day by means of two spirit levels. A computer program was used for monitoring this by comparing left and right leg measurements for each stand.

8. *General Well-Being Schedule:* Each copy of the General Well-Being (GWB) questionnaire was reviewed at headquarters. In addition, every form was checked in the field, and an examiner's observation sheet was filled out giving reasons for not obtaining a full, acceptable GWB. Also included was the interviewer's impression of the degree of comprehension of the interviewee in filling out the GWB.

9. *Laboratory procedures:* Generally, a 10-percent nonrandom sample of blind duplicates was selected for all blood chemistries and serologies. The single exception was the T_3 T_4 determinations for which the lo-percent sample of blind duplicates was chosen in a random fashion. (The nonrandom selection was from the first batch of blood specimens in the first daily session.) The quality control procedures in hematology included the use of Coulter controls. Control results were plotted daily. Blood indices were calculated and used in quality control.

The data collection of the Augmentation Survey was completed in September 1975 with medical histories and household information completed on 94 percent of the 4,288 sample persons; 71 percent of sample persons were examined.

The nonexamined sample persons are of major concern in interpreting the results of the survey. The potential biasing effects of excluding information for nonexamined sample persons are evaluated in the development of each report, and the findings are presented in published reports. In the development of national estimates, imputation procedures to estimate missing data are selected to minimize potential bias in the final results. Imputation procedures used on the data are presented in substantive reports to inform the user of the amount of missing data for which estimated values were substituted and how the values were estimated.

PLANS FOR ANALYSIS AND PUBLICATION OF DATA

Analytical and descriptive reports published by NCHS on HANES findings are usually written by the analytical staff of the Division of Health Examination Statistics, often in collaboration with experts in particular fields.

Before the data are ready for analysis, several preliminary steps must be taken. In some cases, such as reading X-rays, further processing of a data unit is necessary. Data must then be reduced to machine-readable form. A considerable amount of time is usually spent editing data to detect errors in data collection and preparation. For example, examination of cholesterol data in HANES I revealed a large number of greatly elevated cholesterol values in one location. An extra serum vial for these persons was used to repeat the tests; the original values were found to be erroneous, and the repeated tests values were used instead. Editing may also involve comparison of results for variables that are highly correlated, such as body measurements or hematocrit-hemoglobin determinations.

Because of the large amount of data available, it is to be expected that everything cannot be analyzed and published very soon after the end of the survey. Priorities for analyses are governed by such factors as the importance of the data, the necessity of timeliness of publication of particular data, the degree of interest of different groups in the data, and the relative difficulties involved in editing data. Some reports involving the relationships of several data items will require processing of all the involved items before analysis. Most of them should be published in the 5 years following completion of the survey. As in other HES cycles, a set of computer tapes containing the edited data is being prepared for the use of investigators at organizations other than NCHS, for example, universities and other Government agencies. In general, NCHS publishes the results in the Vital and Health Statistics Series 2 and 11 reports. To a lesser extent, information is made available in journal articles and in papers presented at professional meetings.

———— ○ ○ ○ ————

REFERENCES

[1]National Center for Health Statistics: Plan and initial program of the Health Examination Survey. *Vital and Health Statistics*. PHS Pub. No. 1000-Series 1-No. 4. Public Health Service. Washington. U.S. Government Printing Office, July 1965.

[2]National Center for Health Statistics: Plan, operation, and response results of a program of children's examinations. *Vital and Health Statistics*. Series 1-No. 5. DHEW Pub. No. (HSM) 73-1251. Health Services and Mental Health Administration. Washington. U.S. Government Printing Office, Oct. 1967.

[3]National Center for Health Statistics: Plan and operation of a Health Examination Survey of U.S. youths, 12-17 years of age. *Vital and Health Statistics*. PHS No. 1000-Series 1-No. 8. Public Health Service. Washington. U.S. Government Printing Office, Sept. 1969.

[4]National Center for Health Statistics: Plan and operation of the Health and Nutrition Examination Survey, United States, 1971-1973. *Vital and Health Statistics*. Series 1-Nos. 10a and 10b. DHEW Pub. No. (HSM) 7 3-1 310. Health Services and Mental Health Administration. Washington. U.S. Government Printing Office, Feb. 1973.

[5] National Center for Health Statistics: HANES, examination staff procedures manual for the Health and Nutrition Examination Survey, 1971-1973. *NCHS Instruction Manual*, Part 15a. Health Services and Mental Health Administration. Washington. U.S. Government Printing Office, June 1972.

[6]National Center for Health Statistics: Field staff operations manual. *NCHS Instruction Manual*, Part 15b. Health Services and Mental Health Administration. Washington. U.S. Government Printing Office, Sept. 1972.

[7]National Center for Health Statistics: Examination staff procedures manual for the Health Examination Survey, 1974-1975. *NCHS Instruction Manual*, Part 15c. Health Resources Administration. Washington. U.S. Government Printing Office, Apr. 1975.

[8]U.S. Bureau of the Census: Standard metropolitan statistical areas in the United States as defined on May 1, 1967, with populations in 1960 and 1950. *Current Population Reports*. Series P-23, No. 23. Washington. U.S. Government Printing Office, Oct. 9, 1967.

[9]National Center for Health Statistics: Sample design and estimation procedures for a national health examination survey of children. *Vital and Health Statistics*. Series 2-No. 43. DHEW Pub. No. (HSM) 72-1005. Health Services and Mental Health Administration. Washington. U.S. Government Printing Office, Aug. 1971.

[10]Goodman, R., and Kish, L.: Controlled selection-a technique in probability sampling. *J.Am. Stat. Assoc.* 45(251): 350-373, Sept. 1950.

APPENDIXES

CONTENTS

LIST OF APPENDIX TABLES

APPENDIX I

TECHNICAL NOTES ON THE SAMPLE DESIGN

Definition of Terms

Standard metropolitan statistical area (SMSA).-An SMSA consists of a county or group of contiguous counties (except in New England) which contains at least one central city of 50,000 people or more, or "twin cities" with a combined population of at least 50,000 population. In addition, other contiguous counties are included in an SMSA if, according to certain criteria, they are socially and economically integrated with the central city. Definitions of SMSA's which identify the composition and structure of each appear in a U.S. Bureau of the Census publication.[8]

Geographic regions.-For purposes of HES, the 48 contiguous States and the District of Columbia are divided into 4 regions of about the same population size, shown in table I.

Controlled selection.-This term refers to a scheme that permits some element of subjective determination in obtaining a "better balanced" or "more representative" sample, while retaining all the elements of true probability sampling. The procedure is described in a number of publications. [9,10] The control variables used for this sample design are "State groups" and "rate of population change" and are defined as follows:

Separate groups were formed within geographic regions, as shown in table I. To form the State groups, the HIS design strata were classified as belonging to the State in which the HIS sample PSU was located. If a sample PSU was within two States, it was put in the State with the greater proportion of the population.

NOTE: A list of references follows the text.

Table I. State groups by geographic region

Region	State group number	States in group
Northeast	1	New York
	2	Pennsylvania and New Jersey
	3	Maine, New Hampshire, Vermont, Massachusetts, Connecticut, and Rhode Island
Midwest	1	Ohio
	2	Michigan
	3	Indiana and Illinois
	4	Missouri
	5	Kansas, Nebraska, Iowa, and North Dakota
	6	Wisconsin and Minnesota
South	1	Maryland, Delaware, and District of Columbia
	2	Virginia and West Virginia
	3	Kentucky and Tennessee
	4	North Carolina and South Carolina
	5	Georgia
	6	Alabama and Mississippi
	7	Florida
	8	Arkansas, Louisiana, and Texas
West	1	California and Nevada
	2	Texas
	3	Washington, Oregon, Idaho, and Montana
	4	Oklahoma, Arkansas, and Louisiana
	5	Wyoming, Utah, Colorado, New Mexico, and Arizona
	6	North Dakota, South Dakota, Nebraska, Kansas, Minnesota, and Missouri

Rate of population change. -Groups were defined differently for each region as indicated in table II. In the Northeast Region, for example, PSU's with less than a S-percent increase in population between 1950 and 1960 were classified in group 1, while this class in the Midwest

Table II. Ranges for rate-of-population-change control groups by geographic region, 1950-60

Rate-of-population-change group number	Region			
	Northeast	Midwest	South	West
	Percent population change, 1950-60			
1	3 and under	0 and under	-10 and under	-5 and under
2	5-11	1-15	-9-0	-2-0
3	12-23	16-23	1-8	4-21
4	25-58	24-30	9-16	24-39
5		34-81	19-26	40-59
6			27-36	73-167
7			37-47	
8		-	50-301	

Region included only those PSU's with a loss or with no gain in population.

Population density groups. -In general, this term refers to the proportion of the population that lives in urban areas. The density groups are defined somewhat differently for each geographic region.[4] For the very large SMSA's, except those in the South Region, the criterion for inclusion was population size; these SMSA's were chosen for the sample with certainty. In the South Region, the largest SMSA's were defined in the same way as "other large SMSA's," but were put in a different stratum for sampling puposes.

——— *0 0 0* ———

APPENDIX II

SAMPLE LOCATIONS OF THE HEALTH AND NUTRITION EXAMINATION SURVEY OF ADULTS, BY REGION, COUNTY, STATE, AND PROBABILITY DESIGN

Region, county,[1] and State	Probability design		
	1-35	1-65	66400
Northeast			
Essex, Morris, Union, Somerset, Hudson, Middlesex, N.J.	X	X	X
Nassau, Queens, Suffolk, N.Y.	X	X	X
Bronx, N.Y.	X	X	X
Kings, Richmond, N.Y.		X	
Westchester, Rockland, N.Y.: Bergen, Passaic, N.J.		X	
Bucks, Chester, Delaware, Montgomery, Philadelphia, Pa.	X	X	X
Philadelphia, Pa: Camden, Gloucester, Burlington, N.J.		X	
Essex, Middlesex, Norfolk, Plymouth, Suffolk, Mass.	X	X	X
Allegheny, Beaver, Washington, Westmoreland, Pa.	X	X	X
Albany, Schenectady, Rensselaer, Saratoga, N.Y.	X	X	
Lackawanna, Pa.		X	
Holyoke, Chicopee, Springfield, Mass.	X	X	
Bristol, Newport, Providence, Kent, Washington, R.I.		X	
Hartford, Tolland, Conn.	X	X	
Chemung, Tioga, Tompkins, N.Y.		X	
Mercer, Pa.	X	X	
Bedford, Fulton, Pa.		X	
Monroe, N.Y.			X
Blair, Pa.			X
Middlesex, New Haven, Conn.			X
Warren, N.Y.			X
Midwest			
Lake, Porter, Cook, Will, Kane, Ill.	X	X	X
Cook, DuPage, Kane, Lake, McHenry, Ill.		X	
Macomb, Oakland, Wayne, Mich.	X	X	X
Milwaukee, Waukesha, Wis.	X	X	
Hennepin, Ramsey, Anoka, Dakota, Washington, Minn.		X	
Lake, Cuyahoga, Ohio	X	X	
Franklin, Ohio		X	
Buchanan, Mo.	X	X	
Cass, N.Dak.: Clay, Minn.		X	
Jefferson, St. Charles, St. Louis, Mo.: Madison, St. Clair, Ill.		X	
Bay, Mich.	X	X	
DeKalb-Steuben, Ind.: Branch, Mich.	X	X	
Cass, St. Joseph, Mich.		X	
Fayette, Ross, Ohio		X	
LaPorte, Marshall, Starke, Ind.	X	X	
Boone, Greene, Iowa	X	X	

[1]County, parish, or borough.

Region, county,[1] and State	Probability design		
	1-35	1-65	66400
Midwest—Con.			
Howard, Iowa: Fillmore, Minn.		X	
Cass, Clay, Jackson, Platte, Mo.			X
Marion, Ind.			X
Montgomery, Greene, Miami, Ohio			X
Jackson, Mich.			X
Jefferson, Leavenworth, Kans.: Platt, Mo.			X
Brown, Clinton, Ohio			X
Rusk, Wis.			X
South			
St. Bernard, Jefferson, Orleans, La.		X	X
Washington, D.C.: Fairfax, Arlington, Va.: Prince Georges, Montgomery, Md.	X	X	
Richland, Lexington, S.C.	X	X	
Knox, Anderson, Blount, Tenn.		X	
Roanoke, Va.		X	
Chatham, Ga.	X	X	
Hillsborough, Pinellas, Fla.		X	
Palm Beach, Fla.	X	X	
Natchitoches, La.		X	
Lamar, Marion, Miss.	X	X	
Cabarrus, Stanley, Union, N.C.	X	X	
Hancock, Hamblen, Hawkins, Claiborne, Tenn.		X	X
Barbour, Ala.	X	X	
Bullock. Jenkins, Ga.		X	
Sussex, Del.: Worcester, Md.	X	X	
Fayette, W. Va.		X	
Greenville, S.C.			X
New Castle, Del.			X
Jefferson, Ala.			X
Volusia, Fla.			X
Edgefield, Saluda, S.C.			X
Clay, Calhoun, Roane, W. Va.			X
West			
Orange, Los Angeles, Calif.	X	X	X
Los Angeles, Calif.		X	
Alameda, Contra-Costa, San Mateo, San Francisco, Solano, Calif.	X	X	X
Collin, Denton, Dallas, Ellis, Tex.		X	
Bexar, Tex.	X	X	
Pima, Ariz.	X	X	
Douglas, Nebr.: Pottawattamie, Iowa		X	
San Diego, Calif.		X	
Fresno, Calif.	X	X	
Monterey, Calif.		X	
Clallum, San Juan, Wash.	X	X	
Grant, Wash.	X	X	
Gila, Ariz.		X	
Avoyelles, La.	X	X	
Ottertail, Minn.		X	
Adams, Arapahoe, Denver, Jefferson, Boulder, Colo.			X
Sacramento, Calif.			X
Hunt, Rains, Tex.			X
Mason, Thurston, Wash.			X
Greeley, Nance, Nebr.			X
Camadian, Cleveland, Oklahoma, Okla.			X

[1]County, parish, or borough.

QUESTIONNAIRES AND EXAMINATION FORMS

A. Household Card

FORM **HES-5A** (CYCLE IV) 5-15-74	NOTICE — All information which would permit identification of the individual will be held in strict confidence, will be used only by persons engaged in and for the Purposes of the survey, and will not be disclosed or released to others for any purposes.

U.S. DEPARTMENT OF COMMERCE SOCIAL AND ECONOMIC STATISTICS ADMINISTRATION BUREAU OF THE CENSUS ACTING AS COLLECTING AGENT FOR THE U.S. PUBLIC HEALTH SERVICE HOUSEHOLD CARD HEALTH EXAMINATION SURVEY	1. Stand number	2. Identification code	3. Control number			4. Card
			PSU	Segment	Serial	___ of c a r d s

5a. What is your exact address? (Include House No., Apt. No., or other identification and ZIP code)

Listing Sheet

Sheet No. ____

Line No. ____

City	State	ZIP code

b. Is this your mailing address? ☐ Same as 5a
Mark box or specify if different. Include ZIP code.

City	State	ZIP code

c. Special place name | Sample unit number | Type code

6. YEAR BUILT · Ask ➤   ☐ Do NOT Ask

When was this structure **originally** built?

☐ Before 4-1-70   ☐ After 4-1-70 (Go to 8c, complete
(Continue interview)   if required and end interview)

7. Type of living quarters   1 ☐ Housing unit   2 ☐ OTHER unit

8. Area segments ONLY

☐ **a.** Are there any occupied or vacant living quarters besides your own in this building?
    Y (fill Table X)   N

☐ **b.** Are there any occupied or vacant living quarters besides your own on this floor?
    Y (fill Table X)   N

☐ **c.** Is there any other building on this property for people to live in – either occupied or vacant?
    Y (fill Table X)   N

☐ **d.** None

9. Land use   2 ☐ RURAL (Go to 10)   1 ☐ ALL OTHER (19, back)
    ● Regular units coded 82 or 84 in item 2
    ● Special place units coded 82 or 84 in item 2 AND coded 85-89 in item 5c.

10. Do you own or rent this place?   Own ;   Rent ,   Rent for free

11a. Does this place you (own/rent/rent for free) have 10 acres or more? 1 Y   2 N (11c)

b. During the past 12 months did sales of crops, livestock, and other farm products from this place amount to $50 or more?   1 Y (19 back) 2 N (19 back)

c. During the past 12 months did sales of crops, livestock, and other farm products from this place amount to $250 or more?   1 Y   2 N

➤ GO TO QUESTION 19 ON THE REVERSE SIDE

12. What is the telephone number here?   Area code | Number
        None

13. Interviewer's name   Code

➤ NOTE: BEFORE LEAVING **HOUSEHOLD**, CHECK THAT 16 HAS AN ENTRY.
    Determine the best time for callbacks for Supplements and sample persons.

FOOTNOTES

---

14. Noninterview reason

TYPE A
☐ Refusal – Describe in a footnote
☐ No one at home – repeated calls
☐ Temporarily absent – Footnote
☐ Other (Specify) 3
    } Fill items 6-8, 11a-c as applicable 13-15 and 18

TYPE B
☐ Vacant – nonseasonal
☐ Vacant – seasonal
☐ Usual residence elsewhere
☐ Armed Forces
☐ Other (Specify) 7
    } Fill items 6-8, 11a-c as applicable 13-15

TYPE C
☐ Unused line of listing sheet
☐ Demolished
☐ Merged
☐ Outside segment
☐ Built after April 1, 1970
☐ Other (Specify) 3
    } Fill items 8c if marked, and 13-15

15. Record of calls

	Date	Time Beginning	Time Ending	Completed
1		a.m. p.m.	a.m. p.m.	
2		a.m. p.m.	a.m. p.m.	
3		a.m. p.m.	a.m. p.m.	
4		a.m. p.m.	a.m. p.m.	
5		p.m.	a.m.	
6		a.m. p.m.	a.m. p.m.	

16. List line numbers of sample persons not Interviewed during initial Interview.
☐ None

Line number ____

17. Record of additional personal calls

	Date	Time Beginning	Time Ending	Line Nos. completed
1		a.m. p.m.	a.m. p.m.	
2		a.m. p.m.	a.m. p.m.	
3		a.m. p.m.	a.m. p.m.	

NOTE: Footnote reason for noninterviews for sample persons in same detail as in item 14.

18. For "final" Type A noninterviews enter names, approximate ages, and sex of household members.

	Name	Age	Sex
1			
2			
3			
4			
5			
6			

WASHINGTON USE ONLY	Total number of persons	Total number of sampled persons

NCHS Serial Number	Census Use	Name (Last, first) (20a)	How is —— related to —— (head of household)? Relationship (20b)	Household number (20c)	How old was —— on his last birthday? Age (20d)	What is the month, date, and year of ——'s birth? Use card to check birth date and age for consistency. Month / Date / Year (20e)	Enter code W—1 N—2 Ot—3 Race (20f)	Enter code M—1 F—2 Sex (20g)	Is —— now married, widowed, divorced, separated, or never married? M—2 S—6 W—3 N—4 D—5 Marital Status (20h)	Mark (X) the box for all Persons aged 25–74 (20i)	Refer to HES-28 for all EP's to determine if there are any Sample Persons. Enter SP on the line for each Sample Person, then go to HES-5B (20j)
	1			Y N						EP	1
	2			Y N						EP	2
	3			Y N						EP	3
	4			Y N						EP	4
	5			Y N						EP	5
	6			Y N						EP	6
	7			Y N						EP	7
	8			Y N						EP	8
	9			Y N						EP	9
	10			Y N						EP	10

For Office

19a. What is the name of the head of this household? — Enter name in first column.
b. What are the names of all other persons who live here? — List all persons who live here.
c. I have listed (Read names) Is there anyone else staying here now, such as friends, relatives, or roomers?
d. Have I missed anyone who USUALLY lives here but is now away from home?
e. Do any of the people in this household have a home anywhere else?

If any adult males listed, ask:
f. Are any of the persons in his household now on full-time active duty with the Armed Forces of the United States? ..... ☐ Yes → _____ line(s) _____ (Delete) ☐ No

E   If this questionnaire is for an EXTR: unit, enter Control Number of original sample unit _____

TABLE X — LIVING QUARTERS DETERMINATIONS AT LISTED ADDRESS

If in AREA SEGMENT, also enter for FIRST unit listed on property

LISTING SHEET   Sheet number _____   Line number _____

Line No. (1)	LOCATION OF UNIT — Where are these quarters located? Enter exact description or location, e.g., basement, 2nd floor, rear. (2)	• If listed, enter sheet and line number, STOP Table X, and continue interview for original sample unit. • If unlisted, go to 4. (3)	• If outside AREA SEGMENT boundary, mark box below, STOP Table X, and go to Household Page, Item 9; or Medical History, question 1 (as applicable). (4)	USE OR CHARACTERISTICS — Are these (specify location) quarters for more than one group of people? If "yes," fill one line for each group. (5)	OCCUPIED — Do the occupants of these (specify location) quarters live and eat with any other group of people? (6)	ALL QUARTERS Do these quarters in (specify location) have: Direct access from the outside or through a common hall? (7)	Complete kitchen facilities for this unit only? (8)	CLASSIFICATION N — Not a separate unit — Add occupants to this questionnaire. (Complete a separate questionnaire for each unrelated person or family group.) HU — Separate unit; interview on a separate questionnaire. (9)
1		S _ L _	☐ Outside segment boundary	Yes No	Yes — Go to 9 and circle N No	Yes No	Yes No	N HU OT
2		S _ L _	☐ Outside segment boundary	Yes No	Yes — Go to 9 and circle N No	Yes No	Yes No	N HU OT
3		S _ L _	☐ Outside segment boundary	Yes No	Yes — Go to 9 and circle N No	Yes No	Yes No	N HU OT

NOTE — Be sure to continue interview for original sample unit.

B. Sample Person Supplement

FORM **HES-5B** (CYCLE **IV**)
(10-25-74)

U.S. DEPARTMENT OF COMMERCE
SOCIAL AND ECONOMIC STATISTICS ADMINISTRATION
BUREAU OF THE CENSUS'
ACTING AS **COLLECTING** AGENT FOR **THE**
U.S. PUBLIC HEALTH SERVICE

SAMPLE PERSON SUPPLEMENT

HEALTH EXAMINATION SURVEY

Form Approved
O.M.B. No. 68-R1184

NOTICE -All information which would
permit identification of the individual
will be held in strict confidence, will be
used only by persons engaged in and
for the purposes of the survey, and will
not be disclosed or released to others
for any purposes.

a. PSU	b. Segment number	c. Serial number	d. Person number	e. NCHS SERIAL NUMBER

Comments

1. In what State were you born? Enter the name of the State or foreign country.	**1.**	State or foreign country
	(101)	[ ]
2a. What is the highest grade or year of regular school you have ever attended?	**2a.** (102)	o [ ] None Elementary 1 2 3 4 5 6 7 8 High School 9 10 11 12
	(103)	College 1 2 3 4 5+
b. Did you finish the -- grade (year)?	**b.** (104)	1 [ ] Yes 2 [ ] No
3. What is your origin or descent?	**3.** (105)	o [ ] German 8 [ ] Mexican 2 [ ] Italian 8 [ ] **Mexicano** 1 [ ] Irish 7 [ ] Puerto Rican 3 [ ] French 7 [ ] Cuban 4 [ ] Polish 7 [ ] Central or South American 5 [ ] Russian 7 [ ] Other **Spanish** 6 [ ] English 15 [ ] Scottish 12 [ ] **Negro** 15 [ ] Welsh 12 [ ] Black 6 [ ] Mexican-American 15 [ ] Other – **Specify** 7 8 [ ] Chicano
4a. What were you doing MOST of the past **3 months** (For male:): working or doing something else? (For females): keeping house, working, or doing something else?	**4a.** (106)	1 [ ] Working **(4d)** 2 [ ] Keeping house **(4c)** 3 [ ] Something else
b. What were you doing?	**b.** (107)	0 [ ] Layoff 1 [ ] Retired 2 [ ] Student 4 [ ] Ill 5 [ ] Staying home 6 [ ] Looking for work 7 [ ] Unable to work 3 [ ] Other – Specify _____
c. Did you work at a job or business AT ANY TIME during the past 3 months?	**c.** (108)	1 [ ] Yes 2 [ ] No **(5b)**
d. When you were working, did you usually work full time or part time?	**d.** (109)	1 [ ] Full time 2 [ ] Part time
5a. Did you work at any time last **week** or the week **before?** (For females): not counting work around the house?	**5a.** (110)	1 [ ] Yes **(6)** 2 [ ] No
b. Even though you did not work during that time, do you have a job or business?	**b.** (111)	1 [ ] **Yes** 2 [ ] **No**
c. Were you looking for work **or** on layoff from a job?	**c.** (112)	1 [ ] Yes 2 [ ] No **(Instructions for Q-6)**
d. Which – looking for work or on layoff from a job?	**d.** (113)	1 [ ] Looking 2 [ ] Layoff 3 [ ] Both
Ask for all persons with a "Yes" in 5a, b, or c. **If "Yes" in 5c only, questions 6a through 6d apply to this person's LAST full-time civilian job.**	**6a.** For whom did you work? Name of company, business, organization, or other employer.	**6a.** Employer
	b. What kind of **business** or industry is this? For example, TV and radio manufacturing, retail shoe store, State Labor Department, farm.	**b.** Industry (114) [ ][ ][ ]
	c. What kind of work were you doing? For example, electrical engineer, stock clerk, typist, farmer.	**c.** Occupation (115) [ ][ ][ ]
	d. Class of worker (Fill from entries in 60-c; if not clear, read list.)	**d.** (116) 1 [ ] Private paid 2 [ ] Gov. Federal } **(7)** 3 [ ] Gov. other 4 [ ] Own 5 [ ] Nonpaid 6 [ ] Never worked } **(7)**
	If self-employed in "OWN" business and not a farm, ask: **e.** Is the business incorporated?	**e.** (117) 1 [ ] Yes 2 [ ] No

Now I have some questions about your medical history.

7.	Would you say your health in general is excellent, very good, good, fair, or poor?	7.	(118) 1 ☐ Excellent 2 ☐ Very good 3 ☐ Good 4 ☐ Fair 5 ☐ Poor

8a.	Do you have any health problems now that you would like to talk to a doctor about?	8a.	(119) 1 ☐ ✱▯→ 2 ☐ No (9)
b.	What are the problems?	b.	▶DATA PREPARATION USE ONLY◀

(120) 1 ☐ (121) 1 ☐ (122) 1 ☐ (123) 1 ☐
* 2 ☐ * 2 ☐ * 2 ☐ * 2 ☐
3 ☐ 3 ☐ 3 ☐ 3 ☐
4 ☐ 4 ☐ 4 ☐ 4 ☐

9a.	Have you had a cold, flu, or "the virus" during the past month?	9a.	(124) 1 ☐ ✱▯→ 2 ☐ No (IO)
b.	Do you still have it?	b.	(125) 1 ☐ Yes 2 ☐ No

10.	IN THE PAST 5 YEARS have you had a back injury?	10.	(126) 1 ☐ ✱▯→ 2 ☐ No

Now I have some questions about HEARING.

11a.	At any time over the past few years, have you ever noticed ringing in your ears, or have you been bothered by other funny noises in your ears?	11a.	(127) 1 ☐ Yes 2 ☐ No (12)
b.	How often — every few days or less often?	b.	(128) 1 ☐ Every few days 2 ☐ Less often
c.	When it does occur, does it bother you quite a bit, just a little, or not at all?	c.	(129) 1 ☐ Quite a bit 2 ☐ Just a little 3 ☐ Not at all

12a.	Have you EVER had a running ear or any discharge from your ears (not counting wax in the ears)?	12a.	(130) 1 ☐ Yes 2 ☐ No }(13) 9 ☐ DK
b.	How often have you had a running ear or any discharge from your ears?	b.	(131) 1 ☐ Once only 2 ☐ Twice 3 ☐ 3 or more times 9 ☐ DK
c.	Did you visit a doctor because of this condition?	c.	(132) 1 ☐ Yes 2 ☐ No }(13) 9 ☐ DK
d.	Did a doctor give you anything for this condition?	d.	(133) 1 ☐ Yes 2 ☐ No 9 ☐ DK

13a.	Have you EVER had deafness or trouble hearing with one or both ears? Do not include any problems which lasted just a short period of time such as colds.	13a.	(134) 1 ☐ Yes 2 ☐ No (14)
b.	Did you ever see a doctor about it?	b.	(135) 1 ☐ Yes 2 ☐ No
c.	How old were you when you first began having trouble hearing?	c.	(136) 1 ☐ O-4 years old 2 ☐ 5-9 years old 3 ☐ IO-19 years old 4 ☐ 20-29 years old 5 ☐ 30-39 years old 6 ☐ 40—49 years old 7 ☐ 50 years old or older
d.	Since this trouble began, has it gotten worse, better, or stayed about the same?	d.	(137) 1 ☐ Gotten worse 2 ☐ Gotten better 3 ☐ Stayed about the same

e. Was the cause of your hearing trouble or deafness — (Read list)

	Yes	No	DK
Ear infection.	(429) 1 ☐	(430) 1 ☐	(431) 1 ☐
Born with ft. . . . . , , ...	* 2 ☐	* 2 ☐	* 2 ☐
Loud noise such as that from machinery, gunfire blasts, or explosions	3 ☐	3 ☐	3 ☐
Ear surgery . , , ... ✱ .	4 ☐	4 ☐	4 ☐
Ear injury	5 ☐	5 ☐	5 ☐
Other — Specify _____	6 ☐	6 ☐	6 ☐

20

HEARING — Continued

13f. How would you rate your hearing in your RIGHT ear — good, a little decreased, a lot decreased, or are you deaf?

13f. (139) 1 ☐ Good
2 ☐ A little decreased
3 ☐ A lot decreased
4 ☐ Deaf

g. How would you rate your hearing in your LEFT ear — good, a little decreased, a lot decreased, or are you deaf?

g. (140) 1 ☐ Good
2 ☐ A little decreased
3 ☐ A lot decreased
4 ☐ Deaf

h. Have you ever attended d school or class for those with poor hearing or a school for the deaf?

h. (141) 1 ☐ Yes
2 ☐ No

i. Have you ever had any training in lip reading?

i. (142) 1 ☐ Yes
2 ☐ No

j. Have you ever had any training in speech or in speech correction because of poor hearing?

j. (143) 1 ☐ Yes
2 ☐ No

k. Have you ever had any training in how to use your hearing?

k. (144) 1 ☐ Yes
2 ☐ No

l. Have you ever had an operation on your ears?

l. (145) 1 ☐ Yes
2 ☐ No

m. Have you ever had your hearing tested?

m. (146) 1 ☐ Yes
2 ☐ No (13p)

n. How old were you when your hearing was first tested?

n. (147) 1 ☐ 0—9 years old
2 ☐ 10—19 years old
3 ☐ 20—29 years old
4 ☐ 30 years old or older

o. How often do you now have your hearing tested?

o. (148) 1 ☐ Twice a year
2 ☐ Once a year
3 ☐ Once every 2 years
4 ☐ Less often than once every 2 years

p. Have you ever used a hearing aid?

p. (149) 1 ☐ Yes
2 ☐ No (14)

q. Which ear?

q. (150) 1 ☐ Right
2 ☐ Left
3 ☐ Both

r. Do you use a hearing aid now?

r. (151) 1 ☐ Yes
2 ☐ No (14)

s. How well satisfied are you with your present hearing aid? Does it help a lot, a little, very little, or not at all?

s. (152) 1 ☐ Helps a lot
2 ☐ Helps a little
3 ☐ Helps very little
4 ☐ Does not help at all

● If "Yes" in 13p ask 14a—g using the parenthetical phrase "Without a hearing aid."

14a. (Without a hearing aid) Can you usually HEAR AND UNDERSTAND what a person says without seeing his face if that person WHISPERS to you from across a quiet room?

14a. (153) 1 ☐ Yes (15)
2 ☐ No

b. (Without a hearing aid) Can you usually HEAR AND UNDERSTAND what a person says without seeing his face if that person TALKS IN A NORMAL VOICE to you from across a quiet room?

b. (154) 1 ☐ Yes (15)
2 ☐ No

c. (Without a hearing aid) Can you usually HEAR AND UNDERSTAND what a person says without seeing his face if that person SHOUTS to you from across a quiet room?

c. (155) 1 ☐ Yes (15)
2 ☐ No

d. (Without a hearing aid) Can you usually HEAR AND UNDERSTAND a person if that person SPEAKS LOUDLY into your better ear?

d. (156) 1 ☐ Yes (15)
2 ☐ No

e. (Without a hearing aid) Can you usually tell the sound of speech from other sounds and noises?

e. (157) 1 ☐ Yes (15)
2 ☐ No

f. (Without a hearing aid) Can you usually tell one kind of noise from another?

f. (158) 1 ☐ Yes (15)
2 ☐ No

g. (Without a hearing aid) Can you hear loud noises?

g. (159) 1 ☐ Yes
2 ☐ No

The following series of questions will be about specific medical problems or conditions you might have had in the past or might even have at the present time. Please answer "Yes" or "No" to each question.

Have you EVER had —

15a. Pain or aching in any of your joints on most days for AT LEAST 1 MONTH?

15a. (160) 1 ☐ Yes
       2 ☐ No

b. Pain in your neck or back on most days for AT LEAST 1 MONTH?

b. (161) 1 ☐ Yes
      2 ☐ No

c. Pain in or around either hip joint including the buttock, groin, and side of the upper thigh on most days for AT LEAST 1 MONTH?

c. (162) 1 ☐ Yes
      2 ☐ No

d. Pain in or around the knee including the back of the knee on most days for AT LEAST 1 MONTH?

d. (163) 1 ☐ Yes
      2 ☐ No

e. Swelling at a joint, with pain present in the joint when touched on most days for AT LEAST 1 MONTH?

e. (164) 1 ☐ Yes
      2 ☐ No

f. Stiffness in the joints and muscles when getting out of bed in the morning lasting for AT LEAST 15 MINUTES?

f. (165) 1 ☐ Yes
      2 ☐ No

Have you EVER had —

g. Trouble with recurring persistent cough attacks?

g. (166) 1 ☐ Yes
      2 ☐ No

h. A cough first thing in the morning in the winter? (Count a cough with first smoking or on first going out of doors; exclude clearing of throat or a single cough.)

h. (167) 1 ☐ Yes
      2 ☐ No

i. A cough first thing in the morning in the summer?

i. (168) 1 ☐ Yes
      2 ☐ No

j. Any phlegm from your chest first thing in the morning in the winter? (Count phlegm with the first smoke or on going out of doors; exclude phlegm from the nose. Count swallowed phlegm.)

j. (169) 1 ☐ Yes
      2 ☐ No

k. Any phlegm from your chest the first thing in the morning in the summer?

k. (170) 1 ☐ Yes
      2 ☐ No

l. During the past 3 years have you had a period of increased cough and phlegm lasting for 3 weeks or more?

l. (171) 1 ☐ Yes — How many times? 7   2 ☐ No (15m)

(172) 1 ☐ 1 time
    2 ☐ 2 times
    3 ☐ More than 2 times

Have you EVER had —

m. Trouble with shortness of breath, when hurrying on the level or walking up a slight hill?

m. (173) 1 ☐ Yes
      2 ☐ No

n. Wheezy or whistling sounds in your chest?

n. (174) 1 ☐ Yes
      2 ☐ No

o. Trouble with any pain or discomfort in your chest?

o. (175) 1 ☐ Yes
      2 ☐ No

p. Trouble with any pressure or heavy sensation in your chest?

p. (176) 1 ☐ Yes
      2 ☐ No

q. Severe pain across the front of your chest lasting for half an hour or more?

q. (177) 1 ☐ Yes
      2 ☐ No

r. Pains in either leg when walking?

r. (178) 1 ☐ Yes
      2 ☐ No

s. Heart failure, or "weak heart" of any degree of severity?

s. (179) 1 ☐ Yes
      2 ☐ No

t. Infections of the kidneys or bladder?

t. (180) 1 ☐ Yes
      2 ☐ No

u. Loss of vision or blindness lasting from several minutes to several days?

u. (181) 1 ☐ Yes
      2 ☐ No

v. Difficulty in speaking or very slurred speech lasting from several minutes to several days?

v. (182) 1 ☐ Yes
      2 ☐ No

Have you EVER had —

15w.	Prolonged weakness or paralysis of one or both sides of the body lasting up to several months?	15w. (183)	1 ☐ Yes 2 ☐ No
x.	Loss of sensation or numbness or tingling sensations lasting several minutes to several days?	x. (184)	1 ☐ Yes 2 ☐ No
y.	A severe head injury leading to unconsciousness lasting for more than 5 minutes?	y. (185)	1 ☐ Yes 2 ☐ No

► DIABETES

16a.	Do you have any reason to think that you may have diabetes, sometimes called sugar diabetes or sugar disease?	16a. (186)	1 ☐ Yes 2 ☐ No (17)
b.	Did a doctor tell you that you had it?	b. (187)	1 ☐ Yes 2 ☐ No (17)
c.	How long ago did you start having it?	c. (188)	1 ☐ Less than I year ago 2 ☐ I-4 years ago 3 ☐ 5 or more years ago
d.	Do you take insulin shots?	d. (189)	1 ☐ Yes 2 ☐ No
e.	Do you take any medicine by mouth for diabetes?	e. (190)	1 ☐ Yes 2 ☐ No (17)
f.	**What is the name of the medicine?** _____		

► GOITER/THYROID

17a.	Have you ever had a goiter or any other thyroid trouble?	17a. (191)	1 ☐ Yes 2 ☐ No (18)
b.	Who told you that you had goiter or thyroid trouble?	b. (192)	1 ☐ A doctor 2 ☐ A nurse 3 ☐ Other
c.	Is, or was, your thyroid: Overactive (hyperactive) or underactive (hypoactive)?	c. (193)	1 ☐ Overactive 2 ☐ Underactive 3 ☐ Neither 9 ☐ DK
d.	How long ago did you first have this trouble?	d. (194)	1 ☐ Less than I year ago 2 ☐ I-4 years ago 3 ☐ 5-9 years ago 4 ☐ IO or more years ago
e.	Have you been treated by a doctor for goiter or for thyroid trouble?	e. (195)	1 ☐ Yes 2 ☐ No (18)
f.	Were you treated for this condition by a doctor with — (Read list *and mark all that apply*)	f. (196)	1 ☐ Medicines 2 ☐ Surgery 3 ☐ Radiation 4 ☐ Anything else — Specify ↗
g.	Are you currently being treated for this problem?	g. (197)	1 ☐ Yes 2 ☐ No
h.	Are you currently taking any pills or medicine to help you lose or gain weight?	h. (198)	1 ☐ Yes 2 ☐ No
i.	When was the last time you saw a doctor about goiter or thyroid trouble?	i. (199)	1 ☐ Less than I month ago 2 ☐ I-3 months ago 3 ☐ 4-6 months ago 4 ☐ 7-I I months ago 5 ☐ I or more years ago 9 ☐ DK

NOW I would like to ask you some questions about your TEETH.

18a. Have you lost all your teeth from your upper jaw?

18a. (200) 1 ☐ Yes
　　　　 2 ☐ No (19)

b. Do you have a plate for your upper jaw?

b. (201) 1 ☐ Yes
　　　 2 ☐ No (18d)

c. How long have you had your plate?

c. (202) 1 ☐ Less than I year
　　　 2 ☐ I-4 years
　　　 3 ☐ 5-9 years　　　} (19)
　　　 4 ☐ IO-19 years
　　　 5 ☐ 20 or more years

d. Have you ever had a dental plate for your upper jaw?

d. (203) 1 ☐ Yes
　　　 2 ☐ No

e. HOW long has it been since you had any natural or false **teeth** to chew with in your **upper jaw?**

e. (204) 1 ☐ Less than I year
　　　 2 ☐ I-4 years
　　　 3 ☐ 5-9 years
　　　 4 ☐ IO-19 years
　　　 5 ☐ 20 or more years

19a. Have you lost all your teeth from your lower jaw?

190. (205) 1 ☐ Yes
　　　　 2 ☐ No (20)

b. Do you have a plate for your lower jaw?

b. (206) 1 ☐ Yes
　　　 2 ☐ No (19d)

c. How long have you had your plate?

c. (207) 1 ☐ Less than I year
　　　 2 ☐ I-4 years
　　　 3 ☐ 5-9 years　　　} (20)
　　　 4 ☐ 10–19 years
　　　 5 ☐ 20 or more years

d. Have you ever had a dental plate for your lower jaw?

d. (208) 1 ☐ Yes
　　　 2 ☐ No

e. How long has it **been** since you had any natural or false teeth to chew with in your lower jaw?

e. (209) 1 ☐ Less than I year
　　　 2 ☐ I-4 years
　　　 3 ☐ 5-9 years
　　　 4 ☐ IO-19 years
　　　 5 ☐ 20 or more years

● If "Yes" in 18b or 19b ask question 20; otherwise skip to instructions above question 21.

20a. Do you usually wear your plate(s) while eating?

200. (210) 1 ☐ Yes
　　　　 2 ☐ No

b. Do you usually wear your plate(s) when not eating?

b. (211) 1 ☐ Yes
　　　 2 ☐ No

c. Do you usually use **denture** powder or cream to help **keep** your plate(s) in place?

c. (212) 1 ☐ Yes
　　　 2 ☐ No

d. Do **you** think you need a new plate or that the one(s) you have **need(s)** refitting?

d. (213) 1 ☐ No
　　　 2 ☐ Yes, one
　　　 3 ☐ Yes, both
　　　 9 ☐ DK

● If "Yes" to questions 18a and 19a, GO to question 32; otherwise ask:

21. How would **you** describe the condition of your TEETH — **excellent, good,** fair, or poor?

21. (214) 1 ☐ Excellent
　　　 2 ☐ Good
　　　 3 ☐ Fair
　　　 4 ☐ Poor

22. How would **you describe the** condition of your GUMS — xcollent, good, fair, or poor?

22. (215) 1 ☐ Excellent
　　　 2 ☐ Good
　　　 3 ☐ Fair
　　　 4 ☐ Poor

23. How **many times a** day do you usually brush your **teeth?**

23. (216) _____ Times

TEETH — Continued

24. Do you think that you ought to go to a dentist now or very soon for a checkup?   24. | (217) 1 ☐ Yes
No
2 ☐ DK

25. Do you now have an appointment to see a dentist?   25. | (218) 1 ☐ Yes
2 ☐ No

26. Do you think you have any teeth that need filling?   26. | (219) 1 ☐ Yes
2 ☐ No
9 ☐ DK

27a. Do you think you have any teeth that need to be pulled?   27a. | (220) 1 ☐ Yes
2 ☐ No }
9 ☐ DK } (28)

b. Do you think that all of them need to be pulled?   b. | (221) 1 ☐ Yes
2 ☐ No

28a. Have you ever had your teeth cleaned by a dentist or dental hygienist?   28a. | (222) 1 ☐ Yes
2 ☐ No (28c)

b. When was the last time they were cleaned?   b. | (223) 1 ☐ Less than 1 year ago
2 ☐ 1–2 years ago
3 ☐ 3–4 years ago
4 ☐ 5 or more years ago

c. Do you think that your teeth need cleaning now by a dentist or dental hygienist?   c. | (224) 1 ☐ Yes
2 ☐ No
9 ☐ DK

29. Do you have a dentist you usually go to?   29. | (225) 1 ☐ Yes
2 ☐ No

30. How long has it been since you last saw a dentist about yourself?   30. | (226) ☐_____ Months   R
(227) _____ Years (32)
o ☐ Less than 1 month
n ☐ Never (32)

31. Do you go to a dentist AS OFTEN as once every year?   31. | (228) 1 ☐ Yes
2 ☐ No

32a. Do you have an illness which has recently cut down your appetite?   32. | (229) 1 ☐ Yes
2 ☐ No (33)
b. What is the name of the illness? _____

33. Do you have difficulty in swallowing at least 3 days per month? (Don't count the difficulty in swallowing that goes with a cold, sore throat, or flu.)   33. | (230) 1 ☐ Yes
2 ☐ No

34. Have you ever had yellow jaundice (which made your skin or ● yor turn yellow)?   34. | (231) 1 ☐ Yes
2 ☐ No

35a. Have you ever had an abdominal operation for — (Read list and mark all that apply)   35. | (232) 1 ☐ Ulcers
2 ☐ Gal lstones
3 ☐ Hiatus hernia of the diaphragm
4 ☐ Any other condition — Specify ⟍
☐ None

36a. In the past year have you stayed in a hospital overnight or longer?   36a. | (233) 1 ☐ Yes
2 ☐ No (37)
b. For what condition?   b. | ▶DATA PREPARATION USE ONLY◀
(1) First _____ | (234) _____
(2) Second _____ | (235) _____
(3) Third _____ | (236) _____
c. How long were you in the hospital?   c.
(1) First condition . . . . | (237) _____ Weeks
o ☐ Less than 1 week
(2) Second condition . . . . | (238) _____ Weeks
o ☐ Less than 1 week
(3) Third condition . . . . | (239) _____ Weeks
o ☐ Less than 1 week

37a. Has a doctor ever [told] that you had any [of the] following conditio[ns]

● If "Yes" to any of the following conditions, *ask* 37b and 37c for those conditions.

37b. Do you still have it?

37c. How many years ago did you first have it?

Condition		Yes	No	Yes	No	Dk	
Arthritis	(240)	☐	2 ☐	1 ☐	3 ☐	9 ☐	(241) ____
Gout	(242)	☐	2 ☐	1 ☐	3 ☐	9 ☐	(243) ____
Asthma	(244)	☐	2 ☐	1 ☐	3 ☐	9 ☐	(245) ____
Chronic bronchitis or emphysema	(246)	☐	2 ☐	1 ☐	3 ☐	9 ☐	(247) ____
Tuberculosis	(248)	☐	2 ☐	1 ☐	3 ☐	9 ☐	(249) ____
Rheumatic fever	(250)	☐	2 ☐	1 ☐	3 ☐	9 ☐	(251) ____
Heart murmur	(252)	☐	2 ☐	1 ☐	3 ☐	9 ☐	(253) ____
Heart failure	(254)	☐	2 ☐	1 ☐	3 ☐	9 ☐	(255) ____
Heart attack	(256)	☐ (37c)	2 ☐				257 ____
Stroke	(258)	☐ (37c)	2 ☐				259 ____
A peptic, stomach, or duodenal ulcer	(260)	☐	2 ☐	1 ☐	3 ☐	9 ☐	(261) ____
Recurrent or chronic enteritis	(262)	☐	2 ☐	1 ☐	3 ☐	9 ☐	(263) ____
Colitis (spastic colon, mucous colitis)	(264)	☐	2 ☐	1 ☐	3 ☐	9 ☐	(265) ____
Gallstones	(266)	☐	2 ☐	1 ☐	3 ☐	9 ☐	(267) ____
Hepatitis	(268)	☐	2 ☐	1 ☐	3 ☐	9 ☐	(269) ____
Chronic cough	(270)	☐	2 ☐	1 ☐	3 ☐	9 ☐	(271) ____
Pleurisy	(272)	☐	2 ☐	1 ☐	3 ☐	9 ☐	(273) ____
Low blood pressure	(274)	☐	2 ☐	1 ☐	3 ☐	9 ☐	(275) ____
Hay fever	(276)	☐	2 ☐	1 ☐	3 ☐	9 ☐	(277) ____
Allergies to food	(278)	☐	2 ☐	1 ☐	3 ☐	9 ☐	(279) ____
Hives	(280)	☐	2 ☐	1 ☐	3 ☐	9 ☐	(281) ____
Other allergies	(282)	☐	2 ☐	1 ☐	3 ☐	9 ☐	(283) ____
Polio or paralysis	(284)	☐	2 ☐	1 ☐	3 ☐	9 ☐	(285) ____
Hiatus hernia of the diaphragm	(286)	☐	2 ☐	1 ☐	3 ☐	9 ☐	(287) ____
Kidney disease or kidney stones	(288)	☐	2 ☐	1 ☐	3 ☐	9 ☐	(289) ____
Malignant tumor or growth	(290)	☐	2 ☐	1 ☐	3 ☐	9 ☐	(291) ____
Benign tumor, growth, or cyst (except fat or skin)	(292)	☐	2 ☐	1 ☐	3 ☐	9 ☐	(293) ____
Trouble with blood not clotting properly	(294)	☐	2 ☐	1 ☐	3 ☐	9 ☐	(295) 9 __ 5
Nervous breakdown	(296)	☐	2 ☐	1 ☐	3 ☐	9 ☐	(297) ____
Fracture of hip	(298)	☐	2 ☐	1 ☐	3 ☐	9 ☐	299 ____
Fracture of wrist	(300)	☐	2 ☐	1 ☐	3 ☐	9 ☐	301 ____
Fracture of spine	(302)	☐	2 ☐	1 ☐	3 ☐	9 ☐	303 ____
Fracture of any other bone	(304)	☐	2 ☐	1 ☐	3 ☐	9 ☐	305 ____

► ANEMIA

38a. Have you ever had anemia, sometimes called "low blood?"

38a. (306) 1 ☐ Yes
2 ☐ No ⎫ (39)
9 ☐ DK ⎭

b. How long ago did you first have it?

b. (307) _____ Years
oo ☐ Less than 1 year
99 ☐ Don't remember

c. Did a doctor ever tell you that you had anemia?

c. (308) 1 ☐ Yes
2 ☐ No (39)

d. Was the anemia caused by — (Read list)
Poor diet . . . .
Childbirth . . . .
Accidental loss of blood . . . .
Illness . . . .
Surgery . . . .
Any other cause — Specify _____

d.

(432)	(433)	(434) DK
1 ☐	1 ☐	1 ☐
2 ☐	2 ☐	2 ☐
3 ☐	3 ☐	3 ☐
4 ☐	4 ☐	4 ☐
5 ☐	5 ☐	5 ☐
6 ☐	6 ☐	6 ☐

e. Were you treated for this condition by a doctor?

e. (310) 1 ☐ Yes
2 ☐ No (39)

f. Was the treatment you used a — (Read list and mark all that apply)

f. (311) 1 ☐ Better diet
2 ☐ Iron pills
3 ☐ Iron shots
4 ☐ Vitamin pills
5 ☐ Vitamin shots
6 ☐ Transfusions
7 ☐ Any other treatment — Specify ⏋

g. Are you still being treated for this condition?

g. (312) 1 ☐ Yes
2 ☐ No

Now I have some questions about HYPERTENSION

39a. Have you EVER been told by a doctor that you had high blood pressure?

39a. (313) 1 ☐ Yes (39c)
2 ☐ No

b. Another name for high blood pressure is hypertension. Have you EVER been told by a doctor that you had hypertension?

b. (314) 1 ☐ Yes
2 ☐ No (47)

c. About how long ago were you FIRST told by a doctor that you had (high blood pressure/hypertension)?

c. (315) _____ Months
(316) _____ Years
o ☐ Less than 1 month

40. During the past 12 months about how many times have you seen or talked to a doctor about your (high blood pressure/hypertension)?

40. (317) _____ Times
o ☐ None

41. Has a doctor EVER advised you to lose weight BECAUSE OF (HIGH BLOOD PRESSURE/HYPERTENSION)?

41. (318) 1 ☐ Yes
2 ☐ No

42a. Do you now use more salt, less salt, or about the same amount of salt since you learned you had (high blood pressure/hypertension)?

42a. (319) 1 ☐ More
2 ☐ Less
3 ☐ Same

b. Were you EVER advised by a doctor, nurse, or other medical person to use less salt?

b. (320) 1 ☐ Yes
2 ☐ No

43a. Has a doctor EVER prescribed medicine for your (high blood pressure/hypertension)?

43a. (321) 1 ☐ Yes
2 ☐ No (44)

b. Are you now taking any medicine prescribed by a doctor for your (high blood pressure/hypertension)?

b. (322) 1 ☐ Yes
2 ☐ No (44)
3 ☐ No longer has high blood pressure (44)

c. How often are you supposed to take this medicine — more than once a day, once a day, or less than once a day?

c. (323) 1 ☐ More than once a day
2 ☐ Once a day
3 ☐ Less than once a day

d. How often do you take your medicine when you are supposed to — all the time, often, once in a while, or never?

d. (324) 1 ☐ All the time
2 ☐ Often
3 ☐ Once in a while
4 ☐ Never
5 ☐ other — Specify ⏋

HYPERTENSION — Continued

44. ABOUT how many days during the past 12 months has (high blood pressure/hypsrtension) kept you in bed all or most of the day?

44. | 05 — D a y s
o ☐ None

- If "No longer has high blood pressure" in 43b, GO to 45d; otherwise ask:

45a. How often does your (high blood pressure/hypertension) bother you — all the time, often, once in a while, or never?

45a. (326) 1 ☐ All the time
2 ☐ Often
3 ☐ Once in a while
4 ☐ Never (45c)
5 ☐ Other—Specify ➚

b. When it does bother you, are you bothered a great deal, some, or very little?

b. (327) 1 ☐ Great deal
2 ☐ Some
3 ☐ Very little
4 ☐ Other — Specify ➚

- If "All the time" in 45a, GO to 46; otherwise ask:

c. Do you still have (high blood pressure/hypertension)?

c. (328) 1 ☐ Yes (46)
2 ☐ No
9 ☐ DK

d. Is this condition completely cured or is it under control?

d. (329) 1 ☐ Cured (47)
2 ☐ Under control

---

46. Can you tell when your blood pressure is high — that is, do you have any symptoms?

46. (330) 1 ☐ Yes
2 ☐ No

47a. Has a doctor EVER talked to you about problems that con be caused by high blood pressure or hypertension?

47a. 331 1 ☐ Yes (48)
2 ☐ No

b. Has a nurse or other medical person EVER talked to you about problems that can be caused by high blood pressure or hypertension?

b. 332 1 ☐ Yes
2 ☐ No (48)

c. What type of medical person was this?

c. (333) 1 ☐ Nurse
2 ☐ Other — Specify ➚

---

48. ABOUT how long has it been since you LAST hod your blood pressure taken?

48. o ☐ Less than I month
(334) M o n t h s
(335) (___5 Yeats)
77 ☐ Never (51)

---

49. Were you told that your reading was high, low, normal, or were you not told?

49. (336) 1 ☐ High
2 ☐ Low
3 ☐ Normal
4 ☐ Not told
5 ☐ Other — Specify ➚

---

50. During the past 12 months, how manytimes was your blood pressure taken? (Do not count times while a patient in a hospital.)

50. (337) Times

51a. ABOUT how long has it been since you had an electrocardiogram, which involves placing wires on the chest and arms?

51a. o ☐ Less than I year
(338) _____ Years
77 ☐ Never

b. ABOUT how long has it been since you hod o chest X-ray?

b. o ☐ Less than I year
339 — Y e a r s
77 ☐ Never

28

Now, I have some questions about VISION.

52. Are you blind in one or both eyes? 52. �(340) 1 ☐ Yes
2 ☐ No

53a. Do you now have any of the following conditions: Cataracts, glaucoma, detached retina, or any other condition of the retina? 530. �(341) 1 ☐ Cataracts
2 ☐ Glaucoma
3 ☐ Detached retina
4 ☐ Other condition of retina
5 ☐ No condition

b. Do you now have any (other) trouble seeing in one or both eyes even when wearing eyeglasses? b. �(342) 1 ☐ Yes
2 ☐ No

54a. Do you wear eyeglasses? 54a. ⑧(343) 1 ☐ Yes
2 ☐ No

b. Do you wear contact lenses? b. ⑧(344) 1 ☐ Yes
2 ☐ No
- *If BOTH 54a and 54b ore "No," enter B-2 in box in upper right corner and SKIP to Check Item I; otherwise continue with question 55.*

55. How often do you use your (eyeglasses/contact lenses), all of the time, most of the time, some of the time, hardly ever, or never? 55. ⑧(345) 1 ☐ All of the time (*Enter A-I in box in upper right corner and GO to Check Item I.*)
2 ☐ Most of the time
3 ☐ Some of the time
4 ☐ Hardly ever
5 ☐ Never (*Enter B-2 in box and GO to Check Item I.*)

56. Do you use your (eyeglasses/contact lenses) for reading and other close work? 56. ⑧(346) 1 ☐ Yes — A
2 ☐ No — B

57. Do you use your (eyeglasses/contact lenses) for seeing distant objects better? 57. ⑧(347) 1 ☐ Yes —
2 ☐ No — 2

- *If both 56 and 57 ore "No" enter B-2 in the box and ask 58; otherwise record the letter and number from 56 and 57 in the box in upper right corner and GO to Check Item I.*

58. Why do you wear (eyeglasses/contact lenses)?

_____

► CHECK ITEM I ◄

- *If A-I, or A-2, or 8-I is entered in upper right box, READ:*

These first questions ore about how well you can see even when wearing eyeglasses or contact lenses. (Reod the phrase "When wearing **eyeglasses/contact lenses**" in **each** of the following questions.)

- *If B-2 READ:*

These first questions are about how well you con see.

59a. (When wearing eyeglasses/contact lenses) How much trouble do you have seeing with your LEFT eye — a lot of trouble, o little trouble, or no trouble at all? 590. ⑧(348) 1 ☐ A lot of trouble
2 ☐ A little trouble } (60)
3 ☐ No trouble

b. Are you blind in the left eye? b. ⑧(349) 1 ☐ Yes
2 ☐ No

60a. (When wearing eyeglasses/contact lenses) How much trouble do you have seeing with your RIGHT eye — o let of trouble, a little trouble, or no trouble at all? 60a. ⑧(350) 1 ☐ A lot of trouble
2 ☐ A little trouble } (61)
3 ☐ No trouble

b. Are you blind in the right eye? b. ⑧(351) 1 ☐ Yes
2 ☐ No

- *If "Yes" in 59b and 60b, GO to question 62; otherwise ask:*

61a. (When wearing ● eyeglosses/contact lenses) In terms of total vision, how much trouble do you have seeing — a lot of trouble, a little trouble, or no trouble at all? 61a. ⑧(352) 1 ☐ A lot of trouble
2 ☐ A little trouble (62)
3 ☐ No trouble (Check Item II)

b. Are you blind? b. ⑧(353) 1 ☐ Yes
2 ☐ No

620. About how long have you had trouble seeing? 62a. ⑧(354) _____ Months }
⑧(355) _____ Years } (Check Item II)
⑧(356) 1 ☐ Since birth
9 ☐ DK

b. Has it been less than 3 months, or 3 months or more? b. ⑧(357) 1 ☐ Less than 3 months
2 ☐ 3 months or more

► CHECK ITEM II ◄

- If A-I or 6-I in upper right box on page *12,* READ:

  The next questions are about how well you can **see** in recognizing o friend from different distances. (Reod the phrase "When wearing eyeglasses/contact lenses" in *each* of the following questions.)

- If A-2 or B-2 in box, READ:

  The next questions are about how well you can see in recognizing o friend from different distances.

63. (When wearing eyeglasses/contact lenses) Can you SEE well enough to recognize a friend if you get close to his face?	63.	(358) 1 ☐ Yes 2 ☐ No
64. (When wearing eyeglasses/contact lenses) Can you SEE well enough to recognize **o** friend who is an arms length away?	64.	(359) 1 ☐ Yes 2 ☐ No (Check Item III)
65. (When wearing eyeglasses/contact lenses) Can you SEE well enough to recognize a friend across a room?	65.	(360) 1 ☐ Yes 2 ☐ No (Check Item III)
66a. (When wearing eyeglasses/contact lenses) Can you SEE well enough to recognize o friend across a street?	66a.	(361) 1 ☐ Yes 2 ☐ No (Check Item *III*)
b. Do you have any problems seeing distant objects?	b.	(362) 1 ☐ yes 2 ☐ No (Check Item *III*)
c. What types of problems do you have in seeing distant objects? _____	c.	

► CHECK ITEM III ◄

- If A-I or A-2 in the box, READ:

  Now I'm going to ask about how well you con see things that are near to you. Please answer these questions in terms of when you are wearing glasses. (*Read* the phrase "When wearing *eyeglasses/contact* lenses" in each of the following questions where appropriate.)

- If *B-I* or B-2 in box, READ:

  Now I'm going to ask about how well you con see things that are near to you.

67a. Do you reod any newspapers, mogazines, or books?	67a.	(363) 1 ☐ Yes 2 ☐ No (67c)
b. (When wearing eyeglasses/contact lenses) Do you have any trouble at all seeing the print?	b.	(364) 1 ☐ Yes (68) 2 ☐ No (70)
c. Is this because you have trouble seeing?	c.	(365) 1 ☐ Y e s 2 ☐ No
680. (When wearing eyeglasses/contact lenses) Can you SEE well enough to read ordinary newspaper print?	68a.	(366) 1 ☐ Yes (69) 2 ☐ No
b. (When wearing eyeglasses/contact lenses) Con you SEE well enough to recognize letters in ordinary newspaper print?	b.	(367) 1 ☐ Yes 2 ☐ No (69b)
69a. In order to (read/recognize) ordinary newspaper print, must you use a hand magnifying glass?	69a.	(368) 1 ☐ Yes (73) 2 ☐ No (70)
b. Can you see well enough to read or recognize ordinary newspaper print if you use a hand magnifying glass?	b.	(369) 1 ☐ Yes (71) 2 ☐ No (71)
• If 67c is "Yes," GO to 70b; otherwise ask: 70a. Do you have any problem seeing ORDINARY NEWSPAPER print (even when wearing eyeglasses)?	70a.	(370) 1 ☐ Yes 2 ☐ No (73)
b. What types of problems do you have in seeing the print? _____ (73)	b.	
71. (When you are wearing eyeglasses/contact lenses) Can you see large letters in o newspaper, such as the headlines?	71.	(371) 1 ☐ Yes (73) 2 ☐ No
720. If you are in a room, con you see well enough to tell if a light is on or off?	72a.	(372) 1 ☐ Yes 2 ☐ No (73)
b. Can you see welt enough to tell where the light is coming from?	b.	(373) 1 ☐ Yes 2 ☐ No

73. During the past 6 months, have you used any medicine, drugs, or pills internally for the following? (Include any over-the-counter medicine or prescription drugs.) **73.**

		Regularly	Occasionally	No
Sleep problems or insomnia	(374)	1 ☐	2 ☐	3 ☐
Headache.	(375)	1 ☐	2 ☐	3 ☐
Other pains	(376)	1 ☐	2 ☐	3 ☐
Upset stomach or indigestion, ...	(377)	1 ☐	2 ☐	3 ☐
Weak heart	(378)	1 ☐	2 ☐	3 ☐
Allergies.	(379)	1 ☐	2 ☐	3 ☐
Nerves . . . , ...	(380)	1 ☐	2 ☐	3 ☐
Lack of pep (except thyroid pills)	(381)	1 ☐	2 ☐	3 ☐
Convulsions.	(382)	1 ☐	2 ☐	3 ☐
Skin conditions.	(383)	1 ☐	2 ☐	3 ☐
Fluid pills for water loss . . . , ... , . .	(384)	1 ☐	2 ☐	3 ☐
Weight loss (except fluid pills). . , ...	(385)	1 ☐	2 ☐	3 ☐
Infection (antibiotic or sulfa pills or shots only) .	(386)	1 ☐	2 ☐	3 ☐

74a. Are you on a special diet? **74a.** (387) 1 ☐ Yes
               2 ☐ No (75)

b. Is this diet – (Read *list* and mark *all* that apply) **b.**
(388) 1 ☐ To lose weight
*   2 ☐ For diabetes
     3 ☐ For kidney failure
     4 ☐ For ulcers
     5 ☐ For allergies
     6 ☐ For heart' trouble or high blood pressure
(389) 1 ☐ For pregnancy
*   2 ☐ For any other reason – Specify 7

c. Is this diet – (Read list and *mark all* that apply) **c.**
(390) 1 ☐ Low fat
*   2 ☐ Low protein
     3 ☐ Low salt
     4 ☐ Low carbohydrate
     5 ☐ Low calorie
     6 ☐ Some other type – *Specify* 7

d. Was this diet ordered by a doctor? **d.**
(391) 1 ☐ Yes
     2 ☐ No

75. In your usual day, aside from recreation, are you physically very active, moderately active, or quite inactive? **75.**
(392) 1 ☐ Very active
     2 ☐ Moderately active
     3 ☐ Quite inactive

76. In things you do for recreation, for ● xample: sports, hiking, dancing, and so forth, do you got much exercise, moderate exercise, or little or no exercise? **76.**
(393) 1 ☐ Much exercise
     2 ☐ Moderate exercise
     3 ☐ Little or no exercise

These next questions are about the use of TOBACCO.

77a. Have you smoked at least 100 cigarettes during your ● ntire life? **77a.**
(394) 1 ☐ Yes
     2 ☐ No (78)

b. Do you smoke cigarettes now? **b.**
(395) 1 ☐ Yes
     2 ☐ No (77d)

c. On the average, about how many a day do you smoke? **c.**
(396) ___ -Cigarettes per day (77e)

d. How long has it been since you smoked cigarettes fairly regularly? **d.**
(397) ___ -Years (77f)
    77 ☐ Under one year
    88 ☐ Never smoked cigarettes regularly (78)
    99 ☐ DK

77e. On the average, about how many **cigarettes** a day were you smoking 12 months ago?

77e.

(398) Cigarettes per day
88 ☐ Did not smoke
99 ☐ DK

f. During the period when you were smoking the most, about how many **cigarettes** a day did you usually smoke?

f.

(399) Cigarettes per day
99 ☐ DK

g. About how old were you when you first **started** smoking **cigarettes** fairly regularly?

g.

(400) - Years old
88 ☐ Never smoked regularly
99 ☐ DK

78a. Have you smoked at **least** 50 cigars during your entire life?

78a.

(401) 1 ☐ Yes
2 ☐ No (79)

b. Do you smoke cigars now?

b.

(402) 1 ☐ Yes
1 ☐ No

c. About how many cigars a day do you smoke?

c.

(403) _____ Cigars per day (78e)
(IF LESS THAN 1 PER DAY)
88 ☐ 3 to 6 per week (78e)
99 ☐ Less than 3 per week

d. About how long has it **been** since you smoked **three** or more cigars a week?

d.

(404) _____ Years (79)
77 ☐ Under 1 year
88 ☐ Never smoked 3 or more cigars a week (79)
99 ☐ DK

e. **Twelve** months ago, about how many cigars a day did you usually smoke?

e.

(405) - Cigars per day
(IF LESS THAN 1 PER DAY)
77 ☐ 3 to 6 per week
88 ☐ Less than 3 per week
99 ☐ Did not smoke cigars

79a. Have you **smoked at least three** packages of pipe tobacco during your entire **life**?

79a.

(406) 1 ☐ Yes
2 ☐ No (80)

b. Do you smoke a pipe now?

b.

(407) 1 ☐ Yes
2 ☐ No (79d)

c. About how many pipesful of tobacco a day do you usually **smoke**?

c.

(408) _____ Pipesful per day (79e)
(IF LESS THAN 1 PER DAY)
77 ☐ 3 to 6 per week (79e)
88 ☐ Less than 3 per week

d. About how long has it been since you smoked three or more pipesful a week?

d.

(409) _____ Years (80)
77 ☐ Under 1 year
88 ☐ Never smoked 3 or more pipesful a week (80)
99 ☐ DK

e. Twelve months ago, about how many pipesful a day did you smoke?

e.

(410) _____ Pipesful per day
(IF LESS THAN 1 PER DAY)
77 ☐ 3 to 6 per week
88 ☐ Less than 3 per week
99 ☐ Did not smoke a pipe

80. Do you presently use – (Read list and mark all that apply)

80.

(411) 1 ☐ Snuff
2 ☐ Chewing tobacco
3 ☐ Any other form of tobacco -Specify ⟶
☐ None

81.	How important do you think it is for people to have a regular physical check-up, very important, fairly important, or hardly important at all?	81.	④12) 1 ☐ Very important 2 ☐ Fairly important 3 ☐ Hardly important 9 ☐ DK
82.	Is there ONE particular doctor or place you usually go to when you are sick or when you need advice about your health?	82.	④13) 1 • J Yes 2 ☐ No (84)
83.	Where do you go for this care or advice, to a clinic, hospital, doctor's office, or some other place? If Hospital: Is this an outpatient clinic or the emergency room? If Clinic: Is this a hospital outpatient clinic, a company clinic, or some other kind of clinic?	83.	④14) 1 ☐ Private doctor's office 2 ☐ Home 3 ☐ Doctor's clinic 4 ☐ Group practice 5 ☐ Hospital Outpatient Clinic 6 ☐ Hospital Emergency Room 7 ☐ Company or industry Clinic 8 ☐ Other – Specify ↗
84.	How long has it been since you last talked to any doctor about yourself?	84.	④15) – M o n t h s O R ④16) – Y e a r s 0 ☐ Less than 1 month 77 ☐ Never (Check Item IV)
85.	Do you get check-ups from a doctor AS OFTEN as once every 2 years?	85.	④17) 1 ☐ .Yes 2 ☐ No

↗ CHECK ITEM IV ◀

Ask questions 86, 87, and 88 only once for **each family**. If already asked for **this** household, mark (X) the box and end questions. ──────→ ☐

86a.	Is any language other than English frequently spoken here in this home?	86a.	④18) 1 ☐ Yes 2 ☐ No (87)
b.	What language(s)?	b.	Language(s) spoken ④19) ☐
87.	Please look at this card ▬ (Show Flashcard) Which of these Income groups represents yours, your ──'s etc., total combined family **income** for the past **12** months; that is, **since (date)** _____ a year ago? Include income from all sources such as wages, **salaries**, social security or retirement benefits, help from relatives, rent from property, and so forth.	87.	Group ④20) 11 ☐ A 15 ☐ E 19 ☐ I 12 ☐ B 16 ☐ F 20 • J J 13 ☐ C 17 ☐ G 21 ☐ K 14 ☐ D 18 ☐ H 22 ☐ L
88.	May I see your box of table salt?	88.	④21) 1 ☐ Iodized 2 ☐ Not iodized 3 ☐ No box

Comments	
	④22)
	④23)
	④24)
	④25)
	④26)
	④27)
	④28)

C. Water Usage Supplement

FORM HES-SC
(10-24-74)

U.S. DEPARTMENT OF COMMERCE
SOCIAL AND ECONOMIC STATISTICS ADMINISTRATION
BUREAU OF THE CENSUS
ACTING AS COLLECTING AGENT FOR THE
U.S. PUBLIC HEALTH SERVICE

WATER USAGE SUPPLEMENT
HEALTH EXAMINATION SURVEY

a. PSU	b. Segment number	c. Serial number	d. Person number	e. NCHS Serial number

READ - Think of water a person drinks may affect his health. Each house has different water depending on such things as the pipes in the house and the service line to the house. I would like to ask you about your use of drinking water.

• These next four questions are about water and drinks that you make from a faucet at this house. Do NOT include drinks made from water at other locations. 1a. About how many glasses of water do you drink here per day?	1a. 01 _____ glass(es) ☐ ☐ None
b. About how many glasses of cold drinks made from water such as powdered milk, Kool aide, Tang, frozen juice, iced tea, whiskey with water, etc.,do you drink per-day?	b. 02 _____ glass(es) ☐ ☐ None
c. About how many cups of coffee do you drink per day?	c. 03 _____ cup(s) ☐ ☐ None
d. About how many cups of other hot drinks such as tea, soup, etc.,do you drink per day?	d. 04 _____ cup(s) ☐ ☐ None
e. How long have you lived at this address?	e. 05 _____ month(s) 06 _____ year(s)
• Now we have some questions about drinks made from faucets at other locations such as work, restaurants, and so forth. 2a. About how many glasses of water do you drink per day at these places?	2a. 07 _____ glass(es) o ☐ None
b. About how many glasses of cold drinks made from water such as powdered milk, Kool aide, Tang, frozen juice, iced tea, whiskey with water, etc.,do you drink per day?	b. 08 _____ glass(es) ☐ ☐ None
c. About how many cups of coffee do you drink per day?	c. 09 _____ cup(s) o ☐ None
d. About how many cups of other hot drinks such as tea, soup, etc.,do you drink per day?	d. 10 _____ cup(s) ☐ ☐ None

▶ If an entry of glasses or cups in item 2a through d ask questions e and f; otherwise go to item 3.

e. What is the address of the place that you used most in the last month? (Include number, street, city, State, and ZIP code)	e. Address
f. How long have you used water at . . . ?	f. 11 _____ month(s) 113 _____ year(s)

• Now we have some questions about drinks made from **commercial** bottled water. **3a.** About how many glasses of commercial bottled water do you drink per day?	30.	114 _____ glass(es) 0 ☐ None
b. About how many glasses of cold drinks made from **commercial** bottled water such as powdered milk, Kool aide, Tang, frozen juice, iced tea, whiskey with water, etc.,do you drink per day?	b.	(115) _____ glass(es) o ☐ None
c. About how many cups of coffee do you drink per day?	c.	116 _____ cup(s) o ☐ None
d. About how many cups of other hot drinks such as tea, soup, etc.,do you drink per day?	d.	(11) _____ cup(s) o ☐ None

▶ If an entry of glasses or cups in item **3a** through d ask questions **e**, f, and **g**; otherwise to to **item 4.**

e. What brand of bottled water do you use?	a.	Brand name
f. **What** type of water is this (e.g., mineral, distilled, etc.)?	f.	(1)8 1 ☐ Mineral 2 ☐ Distilled 3 ☐ Other (Specify) ↗ _____
g. How long have you used this type of water?	g.	11 _____ month(s) 12 _____ year(s)

• The next questions are about drinks made from other sources such as a well, cistern, spring, etc., on the property but not connected to the house. **4a.** How many glasses of water do you drink per **day?**	40.	121 _____ glass(es) o ☐ None
b. About how many glasses of cold drinks made from **water** such as powdered milk, Kool aide, Tang, frozen juice, iced tea, whiskey with water, **etc.,do** you drink per day?	b.	122 _____ glass(es) o ☐ None
c. About how many cups of coffee do you drink per day?	c.	123 _____ cup(s) o ☐ None
d. About how many cups of other hot drinks such as tea, soup, etc.,do you drink per day?	d.	12 _____ cup(s) o ☐ None

▶ If an entry of glasses or cups in item **4a** through d ask questions e and f; otherwise go to item **5.**

e. What type of source not **connected** to a faucet have you used most in the last month (e.g., well, cistern, spring, **etc.**)	e	125 1 ☐ Well 2 ☐ Cistern 3 ☐ Spring 4 ☐ Other (Specify) ↗ _____
f. Is this source located at home?	f.	126 1 ☐ Yes 2 ☐ No

Ask questions 5 through 10 once for a household. If already asked for this
household, mark (X) the box, end questions and go to Check Item II. ⟶ c I

5.	Does your faucet water come from a public water system or your own water supply?	5.	(127) 1 ☐ No faucet water in structure (10) 2 ☐ Public water 3 ☐ Own supply (7)
5a.	What is the name of the water company that supplies your house?	&a.	(128) Name of company ☐ ☐ ☐
b.	How long have you used water from this company?	b.	(129) _____ month(s) ⎫ (130) _____ year(s) ⎬ (8)
7.	What type of water line runs from your own water supply to the house? Mark (X) one box after reading list.	7.	(131) 1 ☐ Black iron 7 ☐ Cement 2 ☐ Galvanized 8 ☐ Other 3 ☐ Plastic (Specify) ⟋ 4 ☐ Lead _____ 5 ☐ Brass 9 ☐ Don't know 6 ☐ Copper
8a.	Do you have a water softener or conditioner connected to the hot or cold water?	8a.	(132) 1 ☐ Yes 2 ☐ No (9) 9 ☐ Don't know (9)
b.	Which one?	b.	(133) 1 ☐ Hot 2 ☐ Cold 3 ☐ Both 9 ☐ Don't know where connected
c.	What brand is it?	c.	Brand name
9a.	I would like to check the pipes where they are not painted or chrome-plated. May I check under the kitchen sink?	9a.	(134) 1 ☐ Kitchen 2 ☐ At water heater 3 ☐ Other location (Specify) ⟋ _____ (134) 4 ☐ Not checked (Enter reason) ⟋ _____
b.	Mark (X) the type of pipe.	b.	(136) 1 ☐ Black iron 2 ☐ Galvanized 3 ☐ Plastic 4 ☐ Lead 5 ☐ Brass 6 ☐ Copper 7 ☐ Other (Specify) ⟋ 9 ☐ Don't know

36

10.	We will be **analyzing** the water available to **people** for drinking or cooking in their homes. May I take a sample of the water from your kitchen faucet (well, cistern, spring, etc.)?	10.	SAMPLE OBTAINED

10. We will be **analyzing** the water available to **people** for drinking or cooking in their homes. May I take a sample of the water from your kitchen faucet (**well**, cistern, spring, etc.)?

10.

SAMPLE OBTAINED

(137) 1 ☐ Household faucet

2 ☐ Source not **connected** to a faucet

SAMPLE NOT OBTAINED

3 ☐ **Use** bottled water only

4 ☐ Other (Specify) 7

▶ CHECK ITEM II

READ 77-E FOLLOWING:

Thank you very much for answering the questions about **yourself.** To determine more completely and precisely the health status and needs of the adult U.S. population, the U.S. Public Heolth Service also needs actual measurements and tests that can only be obtained **by** a health **examina**tion. For this, a special examination center has been set up and examinations will be conducted on the dates and times indicated on the sheet I will give you. The examination thot is given is very thorough and there are no procedures, such as an internal examination, that ore in **any** way embarrassing.

We very carefully select a sample of people to be representative of all parts of the population. You have been selected from many thousands of people similar to you with respect to your age, **race, and** sex, and the fact that we cannot substitute any other person for you makes **your participa**tion in the examination very important.

The examination is entirely free and you will receive a fee of $10.00 as on expression of appreciation for your help in this important survey and as compensation for your **time and** for any inconvenience. We provide transportation to and from the examination center or we reimburse you if you decide to drive your own car.

None of the results from the examination or answers to the questions I have just asked, will ever be disclosed to anyone for any purpose without the individual's written consent; this is required by law. However, since a valuable examination is being given, most people do request that the examination results be sent to their physician. I would very much like to make an appointment for you at a time that is convenient.

☐ Appointment made
☐ Appointment not made (Specify) 3

Notes

D. Health Care Needs Questionnaire

HRA-11-6 (FORMERLY HSM-411-6)
8-75

Form Approved
O.M.B. No. 68-R1 184

DEPARTMENT OF HEALTH, EDUCATION, AND WELFARE
PUBLIC HEALTH SERVICE
HEALTH RESOURCES ADMINISTRATION
NATIONAL CENTER FOR HEALTH STATISTICS
HEALTH AND NUTRITION EXAMINATION SURVEY

HEALTH CARE NEEDS

a. Name (Lost, first, middle)

b. Deck No.	c. Sample No.	d. Segment No.	e. Serial No.	f. Column No.
181	— — — — —	— — — — —	— —	— —

READ — I need to ask you a number of questions about doctors, dentists, hospitals, and other people who might give you medical core, just how you use them, ond what your opinion is on some questions about health core. Your answers will be kept confidential.

▶ DOCTORS

1. When was the last time you tolked to o doctor obout your own health . .

		Never	Less than 2 weeks ago	2 Weeks through 5 months ago	6 through 11 months ago	1 but less than 2 years ago	2 through 4 years ago	5 or more years ago
at a private doctor's office?	(001)	1 ☐	2 ☐	3 ☐	4 ☐	5 ☐	6 ☐	7 ☐
at a hospital outpatient clinic? . . .	(002)	1 ☐	2 ☐	3 ☐	4 ☐	5 ☐	6 ☐	7 ☐
at a city clinic?	(003)	1 ☐	2 ☐	3 ☐	4 ☐	5 ☐	6 ☐	7 ☐
at a clinic at work?	(004)	1 ☐	2 ☐	3 ☐	4 ☐	5 ☐	6 ☐	7 ☐
ot another type clinic?	(005)	1 ☐	2 ☐	3 ☐	4 ☐	5 ☐	6 ☐	7 ☐
at a hospital emergency room?	(006)	1 ☐	2 ☐	3 ☐	4 ☐	5 ☐	6 ☐	7 ☐
ot home?	(007)	1 ☐	2 ☐	3 ☐	4 ☐	5 ☐	6 ☐	7 ☐
over the telephone?	(008)	1 ☐	2 ☐	3 ☐	4 ☐	5 ☐	6 ☐	7 ☐
in another woy? — Specify _____	(009)	1 ☐	2 ☐	3 ☐	4 ☐	5 ☐	6 ☐	7 ☐

2. What was the MAIN reason for your last visit with a doctor? (Check only one.)

(010)
1 ☐ A sickness or illness --What was the problem? _____

2 ☐ An injury-- Whot was the problem? _____

3 ☐ A follow-up visit
4 ☐ A regular checkup
5 ☐ An injection
6 ☐ For a prescription
7 ☐ Some other reason

3a. For this lost visit, how long was it from the time you decided you should see a doctor until you actually sow him:	3a.	(011) 1 ☐ Less than one day 2 ☐ I-6 days 3 ☐ I but less than 2 weeks 4 ☐ 2-3 weeks 5 ☐ I-2 months 6 ☐ 3 months or more 9 ☐ Don't remember
b. Did you have an appointment to see him?	b.	(012) 1 ☐ Yes – Ask c 2 ☐ No – SKIP to 4
c. How long was it from the time ou made the appointment until you saw I im?	c.	(013) 1 ☐ Less than one day 2 ☐ I–6 days 3 ☐ I but less than 2 weeks 4 ☐ 2-3 weeks 5 ☐ I-2 months 6 ☐ 3 months or more 9 ☐ Don't remember
d. War this time longer thon you would have liked?	d.	(014) 1 ☐ Yes 2 ☐ No 9 ☐ Don't remember
4. From whot place did you leave to go to the doctor?	4.	(015) 1 ☐ From home 2 ☐ From work 3 ☐ From some other place
5. How did you get from there to the doctor?	5.	(016) 1 ☐ Walked 2 ☐ Bus 3 ☐ Own car 4 ☐ Someone else's car 5 ☐ Cab 6 ☐ Ambulance 7 ☐ Other means
6. How long did it take to get there?	6.	(017) 1 ☐ Less than I5 minutes 2 ☐ I5–29 minutes 3 ☐ 30–59 minutes 4 ☐ I hour or mork 9 ☐ Don't remember
7a. At this last visit, about how many minutes did you have to wait before being seen by the doctor?	70.	(018) __ __ __ minutes
b. Do you think this woit was too long?	b.	(019) 1 ☐ Yes 2 ☐ No
8. How well satisfied were you with this visit?	8.	(020) 1 ☐ Satisfied 2 ☐ Not completely satisfied 3 ☐ Dissatisfied 4 ☐ No opinion

9a. During the past 12 months, have you had a health problem which you would have liked to see a doctor about but did not for some reason?

9a.

(021) 1 ☐ *[illegible handwriting]*

2 ☐ No – SKIP to *10*

b. What was the reason you did not see a doctor?

b.

	Yes	No
Lack of confidence in available doctors . . . . (022)	1 ☐	2 ☐
Didn't have time . . . . (023)	1 ☐	2 ☐
Would cost too much. . . . . (024)	1 ☐	2 ☐
Couldn't get an appointment. . . . . (025)	1 ☐	2 ☐
Would have to travel too far . . . . (026)	1 ☐	2 ☐
Didn't have a way to get there . . . . (027)	1 ☐	2 ☐
Was afraid of finding out what was wrong . . . . (028)	1 ☐	2 ☐
Didn't have anyone to care for children or other family members . . . . . (029)	1 ☐	2 ☐
Other – Specify _____ (030)	' c I	2 ☐

_____

10a. When did you last have a general checkup or examination, not counting exams made during a visit for an illness?

10.

(031) 1 ☐ Never – *SKIP* to **13**

2 ☐ Less than 6 months ago

3 ☐ 6–11 months ago

4 ☐ I but less than 2 years ago

5 ☐ 2 years ago of more

9 ☐ Don't remember

11. Where did you get this general examination ?

11.

(032) 1 ☐ Doctor's office

2 ☐ Hospital clinic

3 ☐ Another clinic

4 ☐ Some other place -Specify _____

_____

12. During this lost general examination, were you given –

12.

	Yes	No	
a cardiogram? . . . . (033)	1 ☐	2 ☐	
a blood pressure check? . . . . (034)	1 ☐	2 ☐	
a chest x-ray? . . . . (035)	1 ☐	2 ☐	
blood tests? . . . . (036)	1 ☐	2 ☐	
a urinalysis? . . . . (037)	1 ☐	2 ☐	
vision tests? . . . . (038)	1 ☐	2 ☐	
hearing tests? . . . . (039)	1 ☐	2 ☐	
a rectal examination? . . . . , . (040)	1 ☐	2 ☐	
an internal examination (FEMALES *ONLY*)? . (041)	1 ☐	2 ☐	8 ☐ Not applicable

13a. When was the lost time you received any shots, immunizations or vaccinations to prevent on illness, excluding shots for allergy?

13a. (042)
- 1 ☐ Never – *SKIP* to 14
- 2 ☐ Less than 6 months ago
- 3 ☐ 6-11 months ago
- 4 ☐ 1-2 years ago
- 5 ☐ 3–5 years ago
- 6 ☐ 6-9 years ago
- 7 ☐ 10 years ago or more
- 9 ☐ Don't remember

b. Why did you get this shot?

b. (043)
- 1 ☐ Foreign travel
- 2 ☐ During military service
- 3 ☐ Participation in community or **work**-sponsored immunization campaign (for example, polio or *flu*)
- 4 ☐ Other – Specify _____

14a. Is there o particular doctor you see regularly or whom you would go to if something were bothering you?

14a. (044)
- 1 ☐ ⚕ – ☐ b
- 2 ☐ No – SKIP to 15

b. If you couldn't see this doctor, is there some other particular doctor you would want to see if something were bothering you?

b. (045)
- 1 ☐ Yes
- 2 ☐ No
- 9 ☐ Don't know

15. Except in an emergency, do you need to have on appointment in order to see a doctor?

15. (046)
- 1 ☐ Yes
- 2 ☐ No

16. When you go to o doctor, do you like the doctor to talk to you about your condition or do you like him just to treot it?

16. (047)
- 1 ☐ Talk
- 2 ☐ Just treat

17. Do the doctors you usually see talk to you obout your condition?

17. (048)
- 1 ☐ Yes
- 2 ☐ No

18. Do you try out home remedies or any that you can get without a prescription before going to your doctor about a problem?

18. (049)
- 1 ☐ Yes often
- 2 ☐ Yes, sometimes
- 3 ☐ No

1

NOTES

► DENTIST

19. Do you hove a dentist you usuolly go to?   **19** ⓪③⓪ 1 ☐ Yes   2 ☐ No

20. When wos the lost time you visited or **talked** with o dentist obout yourself. . . . .   **20.**

	Never	Less than 6 months ago	6 through 11 months ago	1 but less than 2 years ago	2 through 4 years ago	5 or more years ago
ot a dentist's office?. . . . . ⓪⑤①	1 ☐	2 ☐	3 0	4 ☐	5 ☐	6 ☐
at a hospital dental clinic? . . . . ⓪⑤②	1 ☐	2 ☐	3 ☐	4 ☐	5 ☐	6 ☐
at o hospital emergency clinic? . . . . ⓪⑤③	1 ☐	2 ☐	3 ☐	4 ☐	5 ☐	6 ☐
ot another clinic (work, school, etc.) . . . . ⓪⑤④	1 ☐	2 ☐	3 ☐	4 ☐	5 ☐	6 ☐
over the telephone? . . . . ⓪⑤⑤	1 ☐	2 ☐	3 ☐	4 ☐	5 ☐	6 ☐
in another way? — Specify ⓪⑤⑥	1 ☐	2 ☐	3 ☐	4 ☐	5 ☐	6 ☐

_____

21. What **was** the MAIN reason for your lost visit or talk with o dentist at either his office or at a clinic?   **21.** ⓪⑤⑦
1 ☐ Adjustment or repair of dental plate
2 ☐ To have a dental plate made
3 ☐ loathache
4 ☐ Tooth pulled or other surgery
5 ☐ Trouble with gums
6 ☐ Regular checkup visit
7 ☐ For cleaning teeth
8 ☐ To have teeth fi l led
9 ☐ For a prescription
o ☐ Some other reason — Specify _____ . -

_____

22. For this last visit, how long was it from the time you decided you needed or wanted to see o dentist until you **actually** saw him?   **22.** ⓪⑤⑧
1 ☐ Less than one day
2 ☐ l–6 days
3 ☐ l week but less than 2 weeks
4 ☐ 2-3 weeks
5 ☐ l-2 months
6 ☐ 3 months or more
9 ☐ Don't remember

23a. At the time of this last visit or talk with a dentist did you have an appointment?	23a.	(059) 1 ☐ Yes – Ask 23b 2 ☐ No – SKIP to 24
b. How long was it from the time you made the appointment until you saw him?	b.	(060) 1 ☐ Less than one day 2 ☐ 1-6 days 3 ☐ 1 week but less than 2 weeks 4 ☐ 2-3 weeks 5 ☐ 1-2 months 6 ☐ 3 months or more 9 ☐ Don't remember
c. Was this wait longer then you would have liked it?	c.	(061) 1 ☐ Yes 2 ☐ No 9 ☐ Don't remember
24. How did you get to the dentist's office?	24.	(062) c ☐ Walked 2 ☐ Bus or subway 3 ☐ Car 4 ☐ Cab 5 ☐ Other means – Specify
25. How long did it take to get there?	25.	(063) 1 ☐ Less than 15 minutes 2 ☐ 15–29 minutes 3 ☐ 30–59 minutes 4 ☐ 1 hour or more 9 ☐ Don't remember
-260. At this last visit with a dentist, about how many minutes did you have to wait before being seen by the dentist?	260.	(064) _ _ _ minutes
b. Do you think this wait was too long?	b.	(065) 1 ☐ Yes 2 ☐ No
27. How well satisfied were you with this visit?	w.	(066) 1 ☐ Satisfied 2 ☐ Not completely satisfied 3 ☐ Dissatisfied 4 ☐ No opinion
28. Does your dentist or dental clinic call you or send you a note to remind you when your next regular checkup is due?	28.	(067) 1 ☐ Yes 2 ☐ No 9 ☐ Don't know
29a. During the past 12 months, have you had a dental problem which you would have liked to see a dentist about but you didn't see the dentist?	29a.	(068) 1 ☐ Yes – Ask 29b 2 ☐ No – SKIP to 30

29b. Why didn't you see bim?

		Yes	No
Didn't have time	(069)	1 ☐	2 ☐
Would cost too much	(070)	1 ☐	2 ☐
Couldn't get on appointment	(071)	1 ☐	2 ☐
Would have to **travel** too for	(072)	1 ☐	2 ☐
Didn't have a **way** to get there	(073)	1 ☐	2 ☐
Didn't have anyone to care for children or other **family** members	(074)	1 ☐	2 ☐
Some other **reason**	(075)	1 ☐	2 ☐

► **HOSPITAL**

30. When **was** the lost time you stayed in a hospital overnight or longer?

(076)
1 ☐ Never – SKIP to 36
2 ☐ Less than I month ago
3 ☐ I-5 months ago
4 ☐ 6-I I months ago
5 ☐ One **year ago or** more
9 ☐ Don't remember

---

31. Was this stay in the hospital on account of on emergency or was it planned in advance?

(077)
1 ☐ Planned
2 ☐ Emergency

---

32. What was the **MAIN reason** you went into the hospital that time?

(078)
1 ☐ Sickness or illness
2 ☐ Injury
3 ☐ Surgery
4 ☐ Child birth ⎫
5 ☐ Checkup   ⎬ **SKIP** to 34
6 ☐ Some other reason – Specify ond SKIP to 34

33a. When you went into the hospital for this _____, just what was the problem?

_____

_____

b. How long was it from **the** time it was decided you needed to go into the **hospital** until you went in?

(079)
1 ☐ Less than one day
2 ☐ I–6 days
3 ☐ I but less than 2 weeks
4 ☐ 2–3 weeks
5 ☐ I-2 months
6 ☐ 3 months or more
s ☐ Don't remember

34a. **What** part of the doctor's bill did you or your family have **to** pay out of your own **pocket** for the treatment the doctor gave you while you were in the hospital?

(080)
1 ☐ None – SKIP to 35
2 ☐ Less than half
3 ☐ More **than** half, but not all
4 ☐ All
s ☐ Don't know – SK/P to 35

b. Did you get any of this money bock from your health insurance?

(081)
1 ☐ Yes
2 ☐ No

35a. What part of this hospital bill did you or your family have to pay out of your own **poc** ket?	**35a.** (082)	1 ☐ None – SKIP to 36 2 ☐ Less than half 3 ☐ More than half, but not all 4 ☐ All 5 ☐ Don't know – 'SKIP to 36
b. Did you get any of this money back from your **health** insurance?	**b.** (083)	1 ☐ Yes 2 ☐ No
36a. **When** you **see** a doctor at his office or at a clinic, **what** part of the cost do you **or** your family usually **have** to pay out of your own pocket?	**36a.** (084)	1 ☐ **Never** been to a doctor – *SKIP to 37* 2 ☐ None – *SKIP* to 37 3 ☐ Less than **half** 4 ☐ More than half, but not all 5 ☐ All 9 ☐ Don't know – *SKIP* to 37
b. Do you get any of this money back from your **health** insurance?	**b.** (085)	1 ☐ Yes 2 ☐ No
37a. Whenever you see o dentist at either his office or at a clinic, what part of the cost do you or your family have to pay out of your own pocket?	**37a.** (086)	1 ☐ Never been to a dentist – *SKIP to 38* 2 ☐ None – *SKIP* to 38 3 ☐ Less than half 4 ☐ More than half, but not all 5 ☐ All 9 ☐ Don't know – *SKIP* to 38
b. Do you get any of this money **back** from your **health insurance?**	**b.** (087)	1 ☐ Yes 2 ☐ No
38a. What part of the cost of drugs **ond** medicines prescribed by your doctor do you **poy** out of your own pocket?	**38a.** (088)	1 ☐ No drugs or medicines ever prescribed – SKIP to 39 2 ☐ None – SKIP **to** 39 3 ☐ Less than half 4 ☐ More than half, but not all 5 ☐ All 9 ☐ Don't know – SKIP to 39
b. Do you get any of this money back from-your health insurance?	**b.** (089)	1 ☐ Yes 2 ☐ No

39. Do you have insurance or **coverage** for medical **care** under . . . .

39b. What **port** of your medical bills **does** it **pay?**

		Yes	No		Less than half	More than **half but** not all	All	Don't know
Medicare (for elderly) ?	(090)	1 ☐	2 ☐	(098)	1 ☐	2 ☐	3 ☐	9 ☐
Private medical insurance?.	(091)	1 ☐	2 ☐	(099)	1 ☐	2 ☐	3 ☐	9 ☐
Insurance through your **place of** work?	(092)	1 ☐	2 ☐	(100)	1 ☐	2 ☐	3 ☐	9 ☐
Medicaid (for all ages) ?.	(093)	1 ☐	2 ☐	(101)	1 ☐	2 ☐	3 ☐	9 ☐
Retired military privileges?. . .	(094)	1 ☐	2 ☐	(102)	1 ☐	2 ☐	3 ☐	9 ☐
Veterans medical care?	(095)	1 ☐	2 ☐	(103)	1 ☐	2 ☐	3 ☐	9 ☐
Some other government assistance program? – Specify _____	(096)	1 ☐	2 ☐	(104)	'cl	2 ☐	3 ☐	9 ☐
Some **other** way?	097	1 ☐	2 ☐	(105)	1 ☐	2 ☐	3 ☐	9 ☐

E. General Well-Being Questionnaire

<table>
<tr><td>H RA-1 I-7 (Formerly HSM-411-7)
/-74</td><td colspan="2">Form Approved
O.M.B. No. 68-R I I84</td></tr>
<tr><td>DEPARTMENT OF HEALTH, EDUCATION, AND WELFARE
PUBLIC HEALTH SERVICE
HEALTH RESOURCES ADMINISTRATION
NATIONAL CENTER FOR HEALTH STATISTICS
HEALTH EXAMINATION SURVEY

GENERAL WELL-BEING</td><td colspan="2">ASSURANCE OF CONFIDENTIALITY
All information which would permit identification of the individual will be held strictly confidential, will be used only by persons engaged in and for the purposes of the survey, and will not be disclosed or released to others for any other purposes (22 FR 1687).</td></tr>
</table>

o. Name (Lost, *first, middle*)	b. Deck No. **171**	c. Sample No. - - - - -	d. Sex 1 ☐ Male 2 ☐ Female	e. Age __ __

READ — This section of the examination contains questions about how you feel and how things have been going with you. For each question, mark (X) the answer which best applies to you.

1. How have you been feeling in general? (DURING THE PAST MONTH)

1. (001)
1 ☐ In excellent spirits
2 ☐ In very good spirits
3 ☐ In good spirits mostly
4 ☐ I have been up and down in spirits a lot
5 ☐ In low spirits mostly
6 ☐ In very low spirits

2. Have you been bothered by nervousness or your "nerves"? (DURING THE PAST MONTH)

2. (002)
1 ☐ Extremely so -- to the point where I could not work or take care of things
2 ☐ Very much so
3 ☐ Quite a bit
4 ☐ Some-- enough to bother me
5 ☐ A little
6 ☐ Not at all

3. Have you been in firm control of your behavior, thoughts, emotions OR feelings? (DURING THE PAST *MONTH*)

3. (003)
1 ☐ Yes, definitely so
2 ☐ Yes, for the most part
3 ☐ Generally so
4 ☐ Not too well
5 ☐ No, and I am somewhat disturbed
6 ☐ No, and I am very disturbed

4. Have you felt so sad, discouraged, hopeless, or had so many problems that you wondered if anything was worthwhile? *(DURING THE PAST MONTH)*

4. (004)
1 ☐ Extremely so -- to the point that I have just about given up
2 ☐ Very much so
3 ☐ Quite a bit
4 ☐ Some -- enough to bother me
5 ☐ A little bit
6 ☐ Not at all

5. Have you been under or felt you were under any strain, stress, or pressure? *(DURING THE PAST MONTH)*

5. (005)
1 ☐ Yes -- almost more than I could bear or stand
2 ☐ Yes -- quite a bit of pressure
3 ☐ Yes -- some - more than usual
4 ☐ Yes -- some - but about usual
5 ☐ Yes - a little
6 ☐ Not at all

6. How hoppy, satisfied, or pleased hove you been with your personal life? (DURING THE PAS7 MONTH)

6. (006) 1 ☐ Extremely happy -could not have been more satisfied or pleased
2 ☐ Very happy
3 ☐ Fairly happy
4 ☐ Satisfied -- pleased
5 ☐ Somewhat dissatisfied
6 ☐ Very di ssati sfi ed

7. Hove you had any reason to wonder if you were losing your mind, or losing control over the way you oct, talk, think, feel, or of your memory? (DURING THE PAS7 MONTH)

7. (007) 1 ☐ Not at all
2 ☐ Only a little
3 ☐ Some-- but not enough to be concerned or worried about
4 ☐ Some and I have been a little concerned
5 ☐ Some and I am quite concerned
6 ☐ Yes, very much so and I am very concerned

8. Have you been anxious, worried, or upset? (DURING THE PAS7 MONTH)

8. (008) 1 ☐ Extremely so -- to the point of being sick or almost sick
2 ☐ Very much so
3 ☐ Quite a bit
4 ☐ Some -- enough to bother me
5 ☐ A little bit
6 ☐ Not at all

9. Hove you been woking up fresh ond rested? (DURING THE PAS7 MONTH)

9. (009) 1 ☐ Every day
2 ☐ Most every day
3 ☐ Fairly often
4 ☐ Less than half the time
5 ☐ Rarely
6 ☐ None of the time

10. Hove you been bothered by any illness, bodily disorder, poins, or fears obout your heolth? (DURING THE PAS7 MONTH)

10. (010) 1 ☐ All the time
2 ☐ Most of the time
3 ☐ A good bit of the time
4 ☐ Some of the time
5 ☐ A little of the time
6 ☐ None of the time

11. Has your doily life been full of things that were interesting to you? (DURING THE PAS7 MONTH)

11. (011) 1 ☐ All the time
2 ☐ Most of the time
3 ☐ A good bit of the time
4 ☐ Some of the time
5 ☐ A little of the time
6 ☐ None of the time

12. Hove you felt down-hearted and blue? (DURING THE PAS7 MONTH)

12. (012) 1 ☐ All of the time
2 ☐ Most of the time
3 ☐ A good bit of the time
4 ☐ Some of the time
5 ☐ A little of the time
6 ☐ None of the time

13. Have you been feeling emotionally stable and sure of yourself? (DURING THE PAS7 MONTH)	13.	(013)	1 ☐ All of the time 2 ☐ Most of the time 3 ☐ A good bit of the time 4 ☐ Some of the time 5 ☐ A little of the time 6 ☐ None of the time
14. Have you felt tired, worn out, used-up, or exhausted? (DURING THE PAS7 MONTH)	14.	(014)	1 ☐ All of the time 2 ☐ Most of the time 3 ☐ A good bit of the time 4 ☐ Some of the time 5 ☐ A little of the time 6 ☐ None of the time

For **each** of the four **scales** below, note that the words ot each end of thq 0 to 10 scale describe opposite feelings. Circle any number along the bar which seems closest to how you have **generally** felt DURING THE PAST MONTH.

15. How concerned or worried about your HEALTH hove you been? (DURING THE PASTMONTH)   15. (015)

0   1   2   3   4   5   6   7   8   9   10

Not concerned at all   Very concerned

16. How **RELAXED** or **TENSE** hove you been? (DURING THE PAS7 MONTH)   16. (016)

0   1   2   3   4   5   6   7   8   9   10

Very relaxed   Very tense

17. How much ENERGY, PEP, VITALITY have you felt? (DURING THE PAST MONTH)   17. (017)

0   1   2   3   4   5   6   7   8   9   10

No energy AT ALL, listless   Very ENERGETIC, dynamic

18. How DEPRESSED or CHEERFUL (DURING THE PAST MONTH) you   18. (018)

0   1   2   3   4   5   6   7   8   9   10

Very depressed   Very cheerful

19. Have you had severe enough personol, emotional, behavior, or mentol problems that you felt you needed help DURING THE PAS7 YEAR?	19.	(019)	1 ☐ Yes, and I did seek professional help 2 ☐ Yes, but I did not seek professional help 3 ☐ I have had (or have now) severe personal problems, but have not felt I needed professional help 4 ☐ I have had very few personal problems of any serious concern 5 ☐ I have not been bothered at all by personal problems during the past year

20. Have you ever felt that you were going to have, or were close to having, a nervous breakdown?	**20.** (020)	1 ☐ Yes – during the past year 2 ☐ Yes -- more than a year ago 3 ☐ **No**
21. Have you ever had a nervous breakdown?	**21.** (021)	1 ☐ Yes – during the past year 2 ☐ **Yes** – more than a year ago 3 ☐ No
22. Have you ever been a patient (or outpatient) at a mental hospital, a mental health ward of a hospital, or a mental health clinic, for any personal, emotional, behavior, or mental **problem**.	**22.** (022)	1 ☐ Yes -- during the past year 2 ☐ Yes -- more than a year ago 3 ☐ No
23. Have you ever seen a psychiatrist, psychologist, or psychoanalyst about any personal, emotional, behavior, or mental problem concerning yourself?	**23.** (023)	1 ☐ Yes – during the past year 2 ☐ Yes – more than a year ago 3 ☐ No

24. Have you talked with or had any connection with any of the following about some personal, emotional, behavior, mental problem, worries, or "nerves" CONCERNING YOURSELF *DURING THE* PAST YEAR?

a. Regular medical doctor (except for definite physical conditions or routine check-ups)	24a. (024)	1 ☐ Yes 2 ☐ No
b. Brain or nerve specialist	b. (025)	1 ☐ Yes 2 ☐ No
c. Nurse (except for routine medical conditions)	c. (026)	1 ☐ Yes 2 ☐ No
d. Lawyer (except for routine legal services)	d. (027)	1 ☐ Yes 2 ☐ No
e. Police (except for simple traffic violations)	e. (028)	1 ☐ Yes 2 ☐ No
f. Clergyman, minister, priest, rabbi, etc.	f. (029)	1 ☐ Yes 2 ☐ No
g. Marriage Counselor	g. (030)	1 ☐ Yes 2 ☐ No
h. Social Worker.	h. (031)	1 ☐ Yes 2 ☐ No
i. Other *formal assistance:*	i. 032	1 ☐ Yes – What kind? _____ 2 ☐ No

25. Do you discuss your problems with any members of your family **or** friends?	**25.** (033)	1 ☐ Yes - and it helps a lot 2 ☐ Yes - and it helps some. 3 ☐ Yes - but it does not help at all 4 ☐ No - I do not have anyone I can talk with about my problems 5 ☐ No - no one cares to hear about my problems 6 ☐ No - I **do** not care to talk about my problems with anyone 7 ☐ No - I do not have any problems

Circle the number for each statement which best describes how often you felt or behaved this way-DURING THE PAST WEEK.

DURING THE PAST WEEK:	Rarely or None of the Time (Less than 1 Day)	Some or a Little of the Time (1-2 Days)	Occasionally or a Moderate Amount of Time (3-4 Days)	Most or All of the Time (5-7 Days)
26. I was bothered by things that usually don't bother me	0	1	2	3
27. I did not feel like eating; my appetite was poor	0	1	2	3
28. I felt that I could not shake off the blues even with help from my family or friends	0	1	2	3
29. I felt that I was just as good as other people .	0	1	2	3
30. I had trouble keeping my mind on what I was doing . . , ...	0	1	2	3
31. I felt depressed.	0	1	2	3
32. I felt that everything I did was an effort . . .	0	1	2	3
33. I felt hopeful about the future	0	1	2	3
34. I thought my life had been a failure	0	1	2	3
35. I felt fearful	0	1	2	3
36. My sleep was restless	0	1	2	3
37. I was happy	0	1	2	3
38. I talked less than usual	0	1	2	3
39. I felt lonely	0	1	2	3
40. People were unfriendly	0	1	2	3
41. I enjoyed life	0	1	2	3
42. I had crying spells	0	1	2	3
43. I felt sad	0	1	2	3
44. I felt that people disliked me	0	1	2	3
45. I could not get "going"	0	1	2	3

46 Filled out by: 1 ☐ Examinee   2 ☐ Interviewer   3 ☐ Mixed

t-IRA-11-7A
12/74

Form Approved
O.M.B. No. 68-R118

EXAMINER OBSERVATION SHEET
(Circle the number for the most appropriate observation for each alphabet set)

47.

A. Test qualifications

   1. Refused at least one item
   2. Couldn't comprehend at least one item
   3. Simple error - missed item, skipped page, etc.
   4. Time called, page missing, other non-examince factor
   5. Feel this is a poor quality record of questionable value (other than above)
   6. Other (describe) ————————————————————
 *7. None - record complete, no qualifications

B. Reasons for not obtaining full, acceptable GWB (assessment limitations)

   1. Lack of interviewers
   2. Lack of time
   3. Examinee failed to return to complete exam
   4. Examinee too ill, drunk, etc.
   5. Foregin language barrier
   6. Seemed to be mentally retarded
   7. Mental functioning or verbal comprehension too limited (o/t 5, 6)
   8. Confused mental state, senile, etc.
   9. Too emotionally disturbed or upset
  10. Refused, non-cooperative, "difficult"
  11. Other (describe) ————————————————————
 * 12. None: obtained full, acceptable GWB

C. Indications of current problems from examinee

   1. Direct reference to a current psychologic problems, i.e., under treatment
      for "nerves", taking tranquilizers, sedatives, sleeping pills, memory loss,
      delusions, senile. brain damage, retarded
   2. Death of someone mentioned as negative affect or distressing
   3. Distressing or limiting medical problem or condition mentioned
   4. Medical or psychologic problem of someone else mentioned
   5. Reference to problems of living, i.e., money, drug use or reaction, alcohol,
      limited physical movement, lonely, unhappy, job loss, unhappy love/sex
      condition, problems with children or spouse, etc.
   6. Reference to problems of other family members, close friends, close
      associates
   7. More than 2 year history mentioned for questions 20-23
   8. Other (describe) ————————————————
 *9. No apparent problems

D. Interviewer impression of subjective distress or state (Any personal, situation,
   or condition mentioned or behavior, appearance, suggesting well being - distress)

   0. Mentally or emotionally disturbed
   1. Severely distressed
   2. Moderately distressed
   3. Mild distress
   4. Some problems but apparently coping well or not distressed
   5. Overly euphoric, hyperactive, or "pushing"
   6. Highly restrained, tense, apprehensive, uncertain
   7. Other (describe) ————————————————
 *8. Mild positive affect (feeling tone or state)
   9. Strong positive affect

E. Interviewer impression of comprehension of task (filling-out GWB)

   0. Could not do task (do not consider negative refusal)
   1. Comprehension low
   2. Comprehension questionable
   3. Translator used or foreign language noted
   4. Literacy level seemed low
   5. Dialect or non-mainstream American-English
   6. Mental processes seemed slow, uncertain
   7. Speech slurred or hardly audible-difficult to understand
   8. Some other problem (describe) ————————————————
 *9. No apparent limitations

NAME: Last, First, Middle

_____

SAMPLE NO. _____

    SEX: M   F

    AGE: _____

48.   GWB examiner number _____
     (If no examiner number, leave blank)

   Comments:

_____

_____

49. Technician Observation

C.

   2.
   3.
   4.

   5.

   6.
   7.
   8.
 *9.

D.

   0.
   1.
   2.
   3.
   4.   Comments:
   5.
   6. _____
   7.
 *8. _____
   9.

E.   _____

   0. 4 _____
   1.
   2. _____
   3.
   4. _____
   5.
   6. _____
   7.
   8. _____
 *9. 50. Technician's Examiner No. _____

51

F. Supplement A—Arthritis

HRA-1 I-2 (FORMERLY HSM-41 I-2)
6-75

Form Approved
O.M.B. No. 68-R1184

DEPARTMENT OF HEALTH, EDUCATION, AND WELFARE

PUBLIC HEALTH SERVICE
HEALTH RESOURCES ADMINISTRATION
NATIONAL CENTER FOR HEALTH STATISTICS

HEALTH AND NUTRITION EXAMINATION SURVEY

SUPPLEMENT A – ARTHRITIS

Name (last, first, middle)	Deck No. 121	Sample No. ____

READ – Earlier you mentioned having had either pain in a joint or in the back or neck, swelling of a joint, or morning stiffness in the joints or muscles. Here are some additional questions about it.

la. Have you had pain in either the back or neck on most days for at least one month?   la. (001)   1 □ ... 2 □ ... 2a

b. Has this pain in the back or neck been present on any one occasion for at least six weeks?   b. (002)   1 □ Yes   2 □ No

c. Where is the pain usually located?   c.

	Yes	No
Neck . . . . (003)	1 □	2 □
Upper back . . . . (004)	1 □	2 □
Mid-back. . . . . (005)	1 □	2 □
Lower back.. . . . . (006)	1 □	2 □

d. When you have this pain, where is it most intense?   d.

	Yes	No
Neck . . . . (007)	1 □	2 □
Upper back . . . . (008)	1 □	2 □
Mid-back. . . . . (009)	1 □	2 □
Lower back. . . . . (010)	1 □	2 □

e. Is the pain present when you are resting at night?   e. (011)   1 □ Yes   2 □ No

f. When you have the pain, does it awaken you from sleep at night?   f. (012)   1 □ Yes   2 □ No

g. Does the pain in the back ever seem to spread?   g. (013)   1 □ Yes   2 □ No   3 □ Not applicable, no pain in back

h. Where does it spread to?   h.

	Yes	No
To the back of the right leg . . . . (014)	1 □	2 □
To the back of the left leg . . . . (015)	1 □	2 □
To the back of both legs . . . . (016)	1 □	2 □
To the top of the head . . . . (017)	1 □	2 □
To the sides of the body . . . . (018)	1 □	2 □

Item I (Continued)

i. Has pain in the neck ever seemed to spread? i.
(019) 1 ☐ Yes
2 ☐ No
3 ☐ Not applicable, no pain in neck

j. Where does it spread to? j.

		Yes	No
To the top and back of the head..........	(020)	1 ☐	2 ☐
To either shoulder area	(021)	1 ☐	2 ☐
To the arms or hands.................	(022)	' c I	2 ☐
Other – Specify_____	(023)	1 ☐	2 ☐

k. Is your back or neck pain made worse – k.

		Yes	No
by coughing, sneezing, or deep breathing?...	(024)	1 ☐	2 ☐
with bending or twisting motion?	(025)	1 ☐	2 ☐
after prolonged activity?	(026)	1 ☐	2 ☐
after prolonged sitting?	(027)	1 ☐	2 ☐
after prolonged standing?.	(028)	1 ☐	2 ☐

l. How old were you when you first experienced this recurring back or neck pain? l.
(029) 1 ☐ Less than 20 years old
2 ☐ 20 – 29 years old
3 ☐ 30 – 39 years old
4 ☐ 40 – 49 years old
5 ☐ 50 – 59 years old
6 ☐ 60 years old or older

m. When was the last time you had this pain? m.
(030) 1 ☐ ☠☐◆
2 ☐ Less than I year ago but not now
3 ☐ I – 2 years ago
4 ☐ 3 – 5 years ago
5 ☐ 6 years ago or more

n. What is the longest episode of back or neck pain you have ever had? n.
(031) 1 ☐ Less than one month
2 ☐ One but less than two months
3 ☐ 2 – 3 months
4 ☐ 4 – 5 months
☐ 6 months or more
9 ☐ Don't remember

o. Does this back or neck pain occur more frequently now than it used to occur? o.
(032) 1 ☐ Yes
2 ☐ No

p. Have you ever had a sprained back due to some type of physical activity? p.
(033) 1 ☐ Yes
2 ☐ ☠☐

q. Have you ever had a "whiplash" injury of the neck? q.
(034) 1 ☐ Yes
2 ☐ No

1r. Hove you ever had a ruptured disc in either your bock or neck?	1r.	035	1 ☐ Yes &'& ◆ 2 ☐ No – SKIP to v
s. At what age?	s.	036	– – years
t. Were you in traction?	t.	(037)	1 ☐ Yes 2 ☐ No
u. Wos surgery necessary?	u.	(038)	1 ☐ Yes 2 ☐ No
v. Hove you ever stayed overnight in a hospital for bock or neck pain?	V.	(039)	1 ☐ Yes 2 ☐ ☒☐

2a. Hove you had pain in or oround either hip joint (including the buttock, groin, and side of the upper thigh) on most days for at least one month?	2a.	(040)	1 ☐ Yes – Ask b 2 ☐ No – SKIP to 3a
b. Has this pain in the hip area been present on any one occasion for at leost six weeks?	b.	(041)	1 ☐ Yes 2 ☐ No
c. Where did you first notice it?	c.	(042)	1 ☐ Left hip 2 ☐ Right hip 3 ☐ Both hips

d. In the hip area, where is the pain usually most intense?

		Yes	No
Right buttock	(043)	'cl	2 ☐
Left buttock	(044)	1 cl	2 ☐
Both buttocks.	045	1 cl	2 ☐
Right groin	046	1 ☐	2 ☐
Left groin	047	1 ☐	2 ☐
Both groins	(048) 048	1 ☐	2 ☐
Side of right thigh	(049)	1 ☐	2 ☐
Side of left thigh.	(050)	1 ☐	2 ☐
Sides of both upper thighs.	(051)	1 ☐	2 ☐
Other – Specify_____	(052)	1 ☐	2 ☐

e. From the hip, has the pain tended to spread to –

		Yes	No
the inside of your leg?	(053)	1 ☐	2 ☐
the front of your leg? . . . . ◢	(054)	1 ☐	2 ☐
the outside of your leg?	(055)	1 ☐	2 ☐
the back of your leg?	(056)	1 ☐	2 ☐

f. Hove you hod pain in or oround the hip when either coughing or sneezing?	f.	(057)	1 ☐ Yes 2 ☐ No
g. When this hip pain is present, does it hurt at rest as well as when moving?	g.	058	1 ☐ Yes 2 ☐ ☒☐

2h. How old were you when you first experienced this recurring pain in the hip?	**2h.** (059)	1 ☐ Less than 20 years old 2 ☐ 20 – 29 years old 3 ☐ 30 – 39 years old 4 ☐ 40 – 49 years old 5 ☐ 50 – 59 years old 6 ☐ 60 years old or older
i. When was the last time you had the pain?	**i.** (060)	1 ☐ Now 2 ☐ Less than I year ago but not now 3 ☐ I – 2 years ago 4 ☐ 3 – 5 years ago 5 ☐ 6 years ago or more
j. What is the longest episode of hip pain you have ever had?	**j.** (061)	1 ☐ Less than one month 2 ☐ ...e but less than 2 months 3 ☐ 2 – 3 months 4 ☐ 4 – 5 months 5 ☐ ...months or more 9 ☐ Don't remember
k. Have you ever had a fractured hip?	**k.** (062)	1 ☐ Yes – Ask I 2 ☐ No – SKIP to p
l. Which hip was broken?	**l.** (063)	1 ☐ Right 2 ☐ Left 3 ☐ Both
m. How old were you when it happened?	**m.** (064)	_ _ Years
n. Was the hip in traction?	**n.** (065)	1 ☐ ☆Ⅲ ◆ 2 ☐ ☒☐
o. Was there surgery?	**o.** (066)	1 ☐ Yes 2 ☐ No
p. Have you ever had o dislocated hip?	**p.** (067)	1 ☐ ☆Ⅲ◆ – ♮& q 2 ☐ No – SKIP to 3a
q. Which hip was dislocated?	**q.** (068)	1 ☐ Right 2 ☐ Left 3 ☐ Both
r. How old were you when it happened?	**r.** (069)	_ _ Years
s. Wos the hip in traction?	**s.** (070)	1 ☐ Yes 2 ☐ No
t. Was there surgery?	**t.** (071)	1 ☐ Yes 2 ☐ No
3a. Have you hod pain in or oround the knee (including the back of the knee) on most days for at least one month?	**3a.** (072)	1 ☐ Yes – Ask b 2 ☐ No – SKIP to 4a
b. Has this pain in the knee area been present on any one occasion for at least six weeks?	**b.** (073)	1 ☐ ☆Ⅲ◆ 2 ☐ No

3c. In which knee did you first have it? 3c.

(074)
1 ☐ Left knee
2 ☐ Right knee
3 ☐ Both knees
9 ☐ Don't remember

d. How old were you when you first experienced recurring pain in the knee? d.

(075)
1 ☐ Less than 20 years old
2 ☐ 20-29 years old
3 ☐ 30-39 years old
4 ☐ 40-49 years old
5 ☐ SO-59 years old
6 ☐ 60 years old or older

e. When this knee pain is present, where is it most intense? e.

	Yes	NO
Right knee..	(076) 1 ☐	2 ☐
☷☓☰ ☖☲☷ ☷☷☷☷☷☷☷☷☷☷☷☷☷☷☷☷	(077) 1 ☐	2 ☐
Both knees	(078) 1 ☐	2 ☐
Behind the right knee	(079) 1 ☐	2 ☐
Behind the left knee	(080) 1 ☐	2 ☐
Behind both knees	(081) ' c I	2 ☐

f. When this knee pain is present, does it hurt at rest as well as when moving? f.

(082)
1 ☐ Yes
2 ☐ No

g. When this knee pain is present, is there also swelling of the knee joint? g.

(083)
1 ☐ Yes
2 ☐ No

h. When this pain is present, have you every had "locking" of the knee? h.

(084)
1 (Yes
2 ☐ No

i. Has either knee ever "given way" under you? i.

(085)
1 ☐ Yes – Ask j
2 ☐ No – SK/P to k

j. Which knee? j.

(086)
1 ☐ Right
2 ☐ Left
3 ☐ Both

k. When was the last time you had this knee pain? k.

(087)
1 ☐ Now
2 ☐ Less than I year ago but not now
3 ☐ I-2 years ago
4 ☐ 3-5 years ago
5 ☐ 6 years ago or more

l. What was the longest episode of knee pain you have ever had? l,

(088)
1 ☐ Less than one month
2 ☐ One but less than 2 months
3 ☐ 2-3 months
4 ☐ 4–5 months
5 ☐ 6 months or more
9 ☐ Don't remember

m. Have you ever hod a fractured knee? m.

(089)
1 ☐ Yes – Ask n
2 ☐ No – SKIP to o

n. Which knee? n.

(090)
1 ☐ Right
2 ☐ Left
3 ☐ Both

56

3o. Have you ever had a severe twisting of either knee with resultant sprain or swelling lasting more than two weeks?	30.	(091)	1 ☐ Yes — Ask p 2 ☐ No — *SKIP* to q	
p. Which knee?	p.	(092)	1 ☐ Right 2 ☐ Left 3 ☐ Both	
q. Have you ever had any other knee injury?	q.	(093)	1 ☐ Yes — Ask r 2 ☐ No — SKIP to 4a	
r. Which knee?	r.	(094)	1 ☐ Right 2 ☐ Left 3 ☐ Both	

4a. Have you ever had hip, knee, or back disease treated by an operation?	40.	(095)	1 ☐ Yes — Ask b 2 ☐ No — SKIP to 5a	
b. Which joint?	b,	(096)	1 ☐ Hip 4 ☐ Hip and knee 2 ☐ Knee 5 ☐ Back and knee 3 ☐ Back 6 ☐ Hip and back 7 ☐ ALL	
IF HIP: (1) Which hip?	(1)	(097)	1 ☐ Right 2 ☐ Left 3 ☐ Both	
IF KNEE: (2) Which knee?	(2)	(098)	1 ☐ Right 2 ☐ Left 3 ☐ Both	
c. What was the operation or procedure? Specify _____				

5o. Have you had pain or aching in any joint other than the hip, back, or knee on most days for at least six weeks?	5a.	(099) 1 ☐ Yes — Ask b and c 2 ☐ No — SKIP to 6a

b. Which joints were painful?   b. & c.

5c. If "Yes," — Which?

	Yes	No		Right	Left	Both
Fingers	(100) 1 ☐	2 ☐	(101)	1 ☐	2 ☐	3 ☐
Wrist	(102) 1 ☐	2 ☐	(103)	1 ☐	2 ☐	3 ☐
Elbow	(104) 1 ☐	2 ☐	(105)	1 ☐	2 ☐	3 ☐
Shoulder	(106) 1 ☐	2 ☐	(107)	1 ☐	2 ☐	3 ☐
Ankle	(108) 1 ☐	2 ☐	(109)	1 ☐	2 ☐	3 ☐
F o o t	(110) 1 ☐	2 ☐	(111)	1 ☐	2 ☐	3 ☐

6a. Have you ever had any swelling of joints with pain present when the joint was touched on most days for at least one month?	6a.	(112) 1 ☐ Yes — Ask b 2 ☐ No — SKIP to 7a
b. Has this swelling been present on any one occasion for at least six weeks?	b.	(113) 1 ☐ ✡ ♏ ✦ 2 ☐ ☆☐

6c. Which joints ore usually involved whenever you have this swelling and tenderness on touching?   **6c. & d.**

	Yes	No	**6d.** If "Yes," – Which?	Right	Left	Both
Fingers...........................	(114) 1☐	2☐	(115)	1☐	2☐	3☐
Wrists.............................	(116) 1☐	2☐	(117)	1☐	2☐	3☐
Elbows ....*.	(118) 1☐	2☐	(119)	1☐	2☐	3☐
Shoulders	(120) 1☐	2☐	0 121	1☐	2☐	3☐
Hips.........	(122) 1☐	2☐	(123)	1☐	2☐	3☐
Knees	(124) 1☐	2☐	(125)	1☐	2☐	3☐
Ankles	(126) 1☐	2☐	(127)	1☐	2☐	3☐
Feet	(128) 1☐	2☐	(129)	1☐	2☐	3☐

6e. How old were you when you first experienced this swelling of the joints?   **e.**

(130)
1 ☐ Less than 20 years old
2 ☐ 20 – 29 years old
3 ☐ 30 – 39 years old
4 ☐ 40 – 49 years old
5 ☐ 50 – 59 years old
6 ☐ 60 years old or older

f. When was the last time you hod this?   **f.**

(131)
1 ☐ Now
2 ☐ Less than I year ago but not now
3 ☐ 1 – 2 years ago
4 ☐ 3 – 5 years ago
5 ☐ 6 years ago or mote

7a. Have you had stiffness in your joints and muscles when first getting out of bed in the morning on most mornings for at least one month?   **7a.**

(132)
1 ☐ Yes – Ask b
2 ☐ No – SKIP to 8a

b. Has this morning stiffness been present on any one occasion for at least six weeks?   **b.**

(133)
1 ☐ Yes
2 ☐ No

c. Which joints are usually involved whenever you have this morning stiffness)   **c. & d.**

	Yes	No	**7d.** If "Yes," – Which?	Right	Left	Both
Fingers............................	(134) 1☐	2☐	(135)	1☐	2☐	3☐
Wrists.............................	(136) 1☐	2☐	(137)	1☐	2☐	3☐
Elbows...........................	(138) 1☐	2☐	(139)	1☐	2☐	3☐
Shoulders	(140) 1☐	2☐	(141)	1☐	2☐	3☐
Hips	(142) 1☐	2;	(143)	1☐	2☐	3☐
Knees	(144) 1☐	2☐	(145)	1☐	2☐	3☐
Ankles...........................	(146) 1☐	2☐	(147)	1☐	2☐	3☐
Feat	(148) 1☐	2☐	(149)	1☐	2☐	3☐
Back.............................	(150) 1☐	2☐				

7e. How long after getting up and moving around does the morning stiffness last?

7e. (152)
1 ☐ Less than 15 minutes
2 ☐ 15 minutes to one half hour
3 ☐ More than one half hour but less than all day
4 ☐ All day

f. How old were you when you first experienced this morning stiffness of joints?

f. (153)
1 ☐ Less than 20 years old
2 ☐ 20 – 29 years old
3 ☐ 30 – 39 years old
4 ☐ 40 – 49 years old
5 ☐ 50 – 59 years old
6 ☐ 60 years old or older

g. When was the last time you had this?

g. (154)
1 ☐ Now
2 ☐ Less than I year ago but not now
3 ☐ I – 3 years ago
4 ☐ 4 – 9 years ago
5 ☐ IO years ago or more

8a. Have you ever had pain, swelling, or stiffness in a joint as the result of an accident or injury?

8a. (155)
1 ☐ Yes – Ask b
2 ☐ No – SKIP to 9

b. Was this the cause of the pain, swelling, or stiffness mentioned previously, do you think?

b. (156)
1 ☐ Y e s
2 ☐ No
9 ☐ Don't know

c. Is this the cause of any pain, swelling, or stiffness which might still be present, do you think?

c. (157)
1 ☐ Yes
2 ☐ No
9 ☐ Don't know

9. Have you ever been treated by any of the following people for your joint troubles?

9.

		Yes	NO
General practitioner.	(158)	1 ☐	2 ☐
Internist , ...	(159)	1 ☐	2 ☐
Rheumatologist	(160)	1 ☐	2 ☐
Orthopedist	(161)	1 ☐	2 ☐
Chiropractor	(162)	1 ☐	2 ☐
Osteopath	(163)	1 ☐	2 ☐
Foot doctor (chiropodist or podiatrist).	(164)	1 ☐	2 ☐
Physical therapist	(165)	1 ☐	2 ☐
Occupational therapist.	(166)	1 ☐	2 ☐
Other – Specify _____	(167)	1 ☐	2 ☐
Never been treated	(168)	9 ☐ SKIP to IIa	

10a. Are you currently being treated by a doctor for the troubles you have just described?

10a. (169) 1 [ ] Yes — Ask *b*
2 [ ] No — *SKIP* to *l lo*

b. What type of doctor is he?

b. (170) 1 [ ] General practitioner
2 [ ] Internist
3 [ ] Rheumatologist
4 [ ] Orthopedist
5 [ ] Chiropractor
6 [ ] Osteopath
7 [ ] Other specialist
8 [ ] Other — *Specify*_____

_____

c. What did he say the problem was?

c.

DATA *PREPARATION USE ONLY*

_____

(171) 1 [ ]   (174) 1 [ ]

_____

(172) 1 [ ]   (175) 1 [ ]

_____

(173) 1 [ ]   (176) 1 [ ]

d. When was the last time you saw him?

d. (177) 1 [ ] Less than l month **ago**
2 [ ] l — 3 months ago
3 [ ] 4 — 6 months ago
4 [ ] 7 — l l months ago
5 [ ] l year ago or more
9 [ ] Don't know

e. Who originally referred you to this doctor?

e. (178) 1 [ ] No one
2 [ ] He's the regular doctor
3 [ ] Another doctor
4 [ ] Family
5 [ ] Clinic
6 [ ] Health nurse
7 [ ] Friend
8 [ ] Other – Specify-.----_____

_____

f. Where do you usually see him?

f. (179) 1 [ ] His office
2 [ ] At a clinic
3 [ ] At home
4 [ ] Other

g. How long will it be until your next visit to him?

g. (180) 1 [ ] Less than l month
2 [ ] l — 2 months
3 [ ] 3 — 6 months
4 [ ] 7 l l months
5 [ ] l year or more
9 [ ] Don't know

11a. Have you ever used any of the following kinds of treatment for your joint troubles?	11a.			11b. Did it do you any good?		
		Yes	No		Yes	No
Splints or casts	(181)	1 [ ]	2 [ ]	(182) 1	[ ]	2 [ ]
. Braces.	(183)	1 [ ]	2 [ ]	(184) 1	[ ]	2 [ ]
Diathermy or paraffin.	(185)	1 [ ]	2 [ ]	(186) 1	[ ]	2 [ ]
Hot packs or heating pads.	(187)	1 [ ]	2 [ ]	(188) 1	[ ]	2 [ ]
Cold packs or ice.	(189)	1 [ ]	2 [ ]	(190)	1 [ ]	2 [ ]
Rest	(191)	1 [ ]	2 [ ]	(192) 1	[ ]	2 [ ]
Traction	(193)	1 [ ]	2 [ ]	(194) 1	[ ]	2 [ ]
Exercises or physical therapy	(195)	1 [ ]	2 [ ]	(196) 1	[ ]	2 [ ]
Aspirin.	(197)	1 [ ]	2 [ ]	(198)	1 [ ]	2 [ ]
Cane	(199) 1	[ ]	2 [ ]	(200)	1 [ ]	2 [ ]
Crutch	(201)	1 [ ]	2 [ ]	(202)	1 [ ]	2 [ ]
Stiff mattress.	(203)	1 [ ]	2 [ ]	(204) 1	[ ]	2 [ ]
Bed board.	(205)	1 [ ]	2 [ ]	(206)	1 [ ]	2 [ ]

c. If "Yes" to 11a or 11b – Do you use it regularly?	c.	Yes	No
Splints or casts	(207)	1 [ ]	2 [ ]
Braces	(208)	1 [ ]	2 [ ]
Diathermy or paraffin.	(209)	1 [ ]	2 [ ]
Hot packs or heating pads.	(210)	1 [ ]	2 [ ]
Cold packs or ice	@ii	1 [ ]	2 [ ]
Rest . . . . :	(212)	1 [ ]	2 [ ]
Traction.. . , , ...	(213)	1 [ ]	2 [ ]
Exercises or physical therapy . . , . , , , . . .	(214)	1 [ ]	2 [ ]
A s p i r i n . . , . . . , ... , . , ...	(215)	1 [ ]	2 [ ]
Cane	(216)	1 [ ]	2 [ ]
Crutch . . . , , ... , , . . .	(217)	1 [ ]	2 [ ]
Stiff mattress, ... , , ... , , ...	(218)	1 [ ]	2 [ ]
Bed board. . , ... , ,	(219)	1 [ ]	2 [ ]

12a. Have you ever had injections into any of your joints?	12a.	(220) 1 [ ] Yes – Ask b
		2 [ ] No -- SKIP to 13a
b. Did they do you any good?	b.	(221) 1 [ ] Yes
		2 [ ] No

13a.	Have you ever taken any of the following medications for your joints?	130.		Yes	No	Don't know
	Any cortisone-like medicine by mouth		(222)	1 ☐	2 ☐	9 ☐
	Butazolidin		(223)	1 c-1	2 ☐	9 ☐
	Darvon or Tylenol. . . , ...		(224)	1 ☐	2 ☐	9 ☐
	Indocin..		(225)	[☐]	2 ☐	9 ☐
b.	If "Yes" – Did it do any good?	b.		Yes	NO	
	Any cortisone-like medicine by mouth		(226)	1 ☐	2 ☐	
	Butazolidin . . . , ...		(227)	1 ☐	2 ☐	
	Darvon or Tylenol. . . . . . . , ... ,		(228)	1 ☐	2 ☐	
	Indocin..		(229)	1 ☐	2 ☐	

14.	Can you do the following things without the help of someone else or the help of some special device?	14.		Yes	No
	Go up or down stairs		(230)	1 ☐	2 ☐
	Get into or out of a car		(231)	1 ☐	2 ☐
	Use washing facilities.		(232)	1 ☐	2 ☐
	Dress yourself		(233)	1 ☐	2 ☐
	Feed yourself , ...		(234)	1 ☐	2 ☐
	Get into or out of bed.		(235)	1 ☐	2 ☐

15.	At the present time, does your joint condition restrict your physical activity very little, quite a bit, or a whole lot?	15.	(236)	1 ☐ Very little 2 ☐ Quite a bit 3 ☐ A whole lot

16.	Have you ever had to stay in bed at home for long periods of time because of your joints?	16.	(237)	1 ☐ Yes 2 ☐ No

17.	Have you ever stayed overnight in a hospital because of joint problems?	17.	(238)	1 ☐ Yes 2 ☐ No

18.	With respect to your joint trouble, would you say your condition is mild, moderate, or severe?	18.	(239)	1 ☐ Mild 2 ☐ Moderate 3 ☐ Severe

19.	What was your job status one month before you first developed your joint condition?	19.	(240)	1 ☐ Retired because of age 2 ☐ Retired because of disability 3 ☐ Unemployed 4 ☐ Working full-time 5 ☐ Working part-time 6 ☐ Housewife with full duties 7 ☐ Housewife with partial or no duties 8 ☐ Other – Specify

_____ - - - A - -

_____ - - - -

20a. As a result of your joint condition, **has** there been a change in your job **status**?	**20a.**	(241) 1 ☐ Yes - A s k *b* 2 ☐ No — *SKIP* to 21
b. What is it now?	**b.**	(242) 1 ☐ Retired because of di sabi li ty 2 ☐ Unemployed 3 ☐ Changed to easier job 4 ☐ Working 5 ☐ Housewife with **partial** duties 6 ☐ Housewife with no duties 7 ☐ Other — Specify _____ _____
21. How many work days do you estimate that you lost during the past 12 months as a result of your joint condition?	**21.**	(243) 1 ☐ None 2 ☐ I — 4 days 3 ☐ 5 — 9 days 4 ☐ 10 — 14 days 5 ☐ I5 — I9 days 6 ☐ 20 — 29 days 7 ☐ 30 days or more
		(244)
		(245)

NOTES

G. Supplement B—Respiratory

<table>
<tr>
<td colspan="2">HRA-11-3 (Formerly HSM-411-3)
4/75

DEPARTMENT OF HEALTH, EDUCATION, AND WELFARE
PUBLIC HEALTH SERVICE
HEALTH RESOURCES ADMINISTRATION
NATIONAL CENTER FOR HEALTH STATISTICS
HEALTH AND NUTRITION EXAMINATION SURVEY
SUPPLEMENT B – RESPIRATORY</td>
<td>Form Approved
O.M.B. No. 68-RI 184

ASSURANCE OF CONFIDENTIALITY
All information which would permit identification of the individual will be held strictly confidential, will be used only by persons engaged in and for the purposes of the survey, and will not be disclosed or released to others for any other purposes (22 FR 1687).</td>
</tr>
</table>

a. Name (Last, first, middle)	b. Deck No. 131	c. Sample No. -----

READ — Earlier you mentioned having had either persistent cough, phlegm, wheezing, shortness of breath, asthma, or hay fever. Here are some additional questions about this trouble.

▶ PERSISTENT COUGHING

Ia. Was your problem that of persistent coughing? Ia.
(001) 1 ☐ Yes – Ask b
2 ☐ No – SKIP to 2a

b. How long have you had this condition? b.
(002) 1 ☐ Less than I year
2 ☐ I-3 years
3 ☐ 4–9 years
4 ☐ IO years or more

c. Have you been bothered by this within the past year? c.
(003) 1 ☐ Yes
2 [No

d. When you have this trouble, do you also have chest pains? d.
(004) 1 ☐ Yes – Ask e
2 ☐ No – SKIP to f

e. Where? e.

	Yes	No
Upper back	(005) 1 ·l	2 ☐
Lower back..	(006) 1 cl	2 ☐
Upperchest.. . . . . • • · ·	(007) 1 ☐	2 ☐
Along the rib edge	(008) 1 ☐	2 ☐
On the sides . . . . . , ... , . . .	(009) 1 ☐	2 ☐

f. Do you bring up phlegm with the cough? f.
(010) 1 ☐ Yes
2 ☐ No

g. Do you cough persistently like this on most days for as much as. THREE months each year? g.
(011) 1 ☐ Yes
2 ☐ No

h. Do any medicines you take help relieve the cough? h.
(012) 1 ☐ Yes
2 ☐ No

i. What time of year do these coughing attacks seem at their worst? i.
(013) 1 ☐ Winter
2 ☐ Summer
3 ☐ No difference

2a.	Have you had trouble with coughing spells when you first get up in the early morning? (Count a cough with first smoke or on first going out of doors; exclude clearing of throat or a single cough.)	**2a.**	(014) 1 ☐ Yes — Ask b 2 ☐ No — SKIP to 3a
b.	**How** long have you had this particular condition?	**b.**	(015) 1 ☐ Less than I year 2 ☐ I-3 years 3 ☐ 4-9 years 4 ☐ 10 years or more 9 ☐ Don't know
c.	Do you have chest pains when you have morning coughing spells?	**c.**	(016) 1 ☐ Yes — Ask d 2 ☐ No — SKIP to e
d.	Where?	**d.**	Yes No
	Upper **back** . . . . , ...		(017) 1 ☐ 2 ☐
	Lower back..		(018) 1 ☐ 2 ☐
	Upper chest.		(019) 1 ☐ 2 ☐
	Along the rib edge.		(020) 1 ☐ 2 ☐
	On the sides		(021) 1 ☐ 2 ☐
e.	What time of year are these morning coughing spells at their worst?	**e.**	(022) 1 ☐ Winter 2 ☐ Summer 3 ☐ No difference
f.	Do you have a morning cough like this on most days for as much as **THREE** months each year?	**f.**	(023) 1 ☐ Yes 2 ☐ No
g.	Do you usually have a persistent cough at other times during the day or at night in the winter? (**IGNORE** AN OCCASIONAL COUGH.)	**g.**	(024) 1 ☐ Yes 2 ☐ No
h.	Do you usually have a persistent cough at other times during the day or at night in the summer? (IGNORE AN OCCASIONAL COUGH.)	**h.**	(025) 1 ☐ Yes 2 ☐ No

▶ PHLEGM

3a.	Do you usually bring up any phlegm from your chest first thing in the morning? (Count phelgm with the first smoke or on going out of doors. Exclude phlegm from the nose. Count swallowed phlegm.)	30.	(026) 1 ☐ Yes — Ask b 2 ☐ No — SKIP to 4a
b.	How long have you had this condition?	**b.**	(027) 1 ☐ Less than I year 2 ☐ I-3 years 3 ☐ 4-9 years 4 ☐ 10 years or more 9 ☐ Don't know

		Yes	No
c. What color is the phlegm?	c.		
Green.	(028)	1 ☐	2 ☐
Yellow.	(029)	1 ☐	2 ☐
Clear	(030)	1 ☐	2 ☐
Blood-streaked.	(031)	1 ☐	2 ☐

d. Do you also bring up any phlegm from your chest at other times during the day or at night, in the winter? (At *least* two times or more)

d. (032) 1 ☐ Yes
      2 ☐ No

e. Do you also bring up any phlegm from your chest during the day, or at night, in the summer? (At *least* two *times* or more)

e. (033) 1 (Y e s
      2 ☐ No

f. What time of year do you seem to bring up the most phlegm from your chest?

f. (034) 1 ☐ Winter
      2 ☐ Summer
      3 ☐ No difference

g. If you have brought up phlegm, do you bring it up on most days for as much as THREE months each year?

g. (035) 1 ☐ Y e s
      2 ☐ No

▶ SHORTNESS OF BREATH

4a. Have you had shortness of breath either when hurrying on the level or walking up ,a slight hill?

4a. (036) 1 ☐ ✡ℳ♦ — Ask b
      2 ☐ No – SKIP to 5a

b. Have you had this problem most days for as much as THREE months'each year?

b. (037) ☐ ✡ℳ♦
      2 ☐ No

c. Do you get short of breath when walking with other people at an ordinary pace on the level?

c. (038) 1 ☐ Yes
      2 ☐ No

d. Do you have to stop for breath when walking at your own pace on the level?

d. (039) 1 ☐ Yes
      2 ☐ No

e. Do you have to stop for breath after walking about 100 yards or after a few minutes on the level?

e. (040) 1 ☐ Yes
      2 ☐ ✂☐

f. How long ago did you first have this trouble with shortness of breath?

f. (041) 1 ☐ Less than I year ago
      2 ☐ I-3 **years** ago
      3 ☐ **4-9 years** ago
      4 ☐ IO years ago or more
      9 ☐ Don't know

g. Have you gotten chest pains along with the shortness of breath?

g. (042) 1 ☐ Y e s – Ask h
      2 ☐ No – *SKIP* to i

		Yes	No
h. Where?	h.		
Upper chest.	(043)	1 ☐	2 ☐
Upper back . . . . , ... , ...	(044)	1 ☐	2 ☐
Lower back.. . . . , , ...	(045)	1 ☐	2 ☐
Along the lower ribs	(046)	1 ☐	2 ☐
On the sides	(047)	1 ☐	2 ☐

4i. Do you develop wheezing as well as shortness of breath?	4i.	(048)	1 ☐ ☆ ♍ ♦ 2 ☐ ☠ ☐
j. Have you ever felt like you were going to pass out from the shortness of breath?	j.	(049)	1 ☐ Yes 2 ☐ No

► WHEEZING

5a. Has your chest ever sounded wheezy or whistling?	5a.	(050)	1 ☐ Yes — Ask b 2 ☐ No — SKIP to 6a
b. How long have you had this condition?	b.	(051)	1 ☐ Less than I year 2 ☐ I-3 years 3 ☐ 4-9 years 4 ☐ IO years or more
c. Do you get this wheezing or whistling with colds?	c.	(052)	1 ☐ Yes 2 ☐ No
d. Do you get this occasionally apart from colds?	d.	(053)	1 ☐ Yes 2 ☐ No
e. Does this usually occur daily?	e.	(054)	1 ☐ Yes 2 ☐ No
f. What time of year does it seem worst?	f.	(055)	1 ☐ Winter 2 ☐ Summer 3 ☐ No difference
g. Is this wheeziness present on most days for as much as THREE months each year?	g.	(056)	1 ☐ ☆♍ ♦ 2 ☐ ☠ ☐
h. Do you take any medicines for wheezing?	h.	(057)	1 ☐ Yes — Ask i 2 ☐ No — SKIP to 6a
i. Do they help relieve the wheezing?	i.	(058)	1 ☐ Not at all 2 ☐ A small amount 3 ☐ A great deal

► ASTHMA

6a. Have you had, or do you now have asthma?	6a.	(059)	1 ☐ Yes — Ask b 2 ☐ No — SKIP to 7a

b. What is it related to or due to?	b.		Yes	No
Dust		(060)	1 ☐	2 ☐
Foods		(061)	1 ☐	2 ☐
Animal contacts		(062)	1 ☐	2 ☐
Drugs		(063)	1 ☐	2 ☐
Pollens		(064)	1 ☐	2 ☐
Molds		(065)	1 ☐	2 ☐
Other — Specify ———————		(066)	1 ☐	2 ☐
Don't know		(067)	9 ☐	

6c. How long have you had this condition?   **6c.**

(068)
- 1 ☐ Less than 1 year – *SKIP* to e
- 2 ☐ 1–3 years – *SKIP* to e
- 3 ☐ 4–9 years ago – *SKIP* to e
- 4 ☐ 10 years or more – Go to *d*

d, Since you were a child?   **d.**

(069)
- 1 ☐ Yes
- 2 ☐ No

e. Do you have asthma symptoms on most days for as much as THREE months each year?   **e.**

(070)
- 1 ☐ Yes
- 2 ☐ No

f. What time of year is it worst?   **f.**

	Yes	No
Spring . . . . (071)	1 ☐	2 ☐
Summer . . . . (072)	1 ☐	2 ☐
Fall . . . . (073)	☐	2 ☐
Winter . . . . (074)	1 ☐	2 ☐

g. Do you take any medicines for it?   **g.**

(075)
- 1 ☐ Yes
- 2 ☐ No

▶ **HAYFEVER**

7a. Have you had, or do you now have, hayfever?   **7a.**

(076)
- 1 ☐ Yes – Ask b
- 2 ☐ No – SKIP to 8*a*

b. What is it related to or due to?   **b.**

	Yes	No
Dust . . . . (077)	1 ☐	2 ☐
Foods . . . . (078)	1 ☐	2 ☐
Animal contacts . . . , ... (079)	1 ☐	2 ☐
Drugs . . . . (080)	c 1	2 ☐
Pollens.. . . . . , ... (081)	1 ☐	2 ☐
Molds . . . . (082)	1 ☐	2 ☐
Air conditioners . . . . (083)	1 ☐	2 ☐
Other – Specify _____ (084)	1 ☐	2 ☐
Don't know . . . . , , , (085)	9 ☐	

c* How long have you had this condition?   **c.**

(086)
- 1 ☐ Less than 1 year – SKIP to e
- 2 ☐ 1-3 years – SKIP to e
- 3 ☐ 4–9 years – SKIP to e
- 4 ☐ 10 years or more – Ask *d*

d. Since you were a child?   **d.**

(087)
- 1 ☐ Yes
- 2 ☐ No

68

7e. Do you have **hayfever** symptoms on most days for as much as THREE months each year?	7e.	(088) 1 ☐ Yes 2 ☐ No

f. What time of the year is it worst? f.

		Yes	No
Spring..	(089)	1 ☐	2 ☐
Summer.	(090)	1 ☐	2 ☐
Fall . . . . • • • . . . • • •	(091)	c I	2 ☐
Winter	(092)	1 ☐	2 ☐

g. Do you take any medicines for it? g. (093) 1 ☐ Yes
2 ☐ No

► MEDICAL CARE

8a. Have you ever been tested for TB (tuberculosis)? | 8a. | (094) 1 ☐ Yes — Ask b
2 ☐ No — SKIP to 9a

b. How were you tested? b.

		Yes	No
A skin test . . . . , . .	(095)	c I	2 ☐
Chest **x-ray** . . . , ... • . • . . .	(096)	1 ☐	2 ☐
Sputum examination	(097)	E I	2 ☐
Don't know	(098)	9 c I	

c. How often are you tested? c. (099) 1 ☐ Once every year
2 ☐ Once every two years
3 ☐ Once every 3-5 years
4 ☐ Less often than once every 5 years

d. How long ago were you last tested? d. (100) 1 ☐ Less than I year ago
2 ☐ I-2 years ago
3 ☐ 3-5 years ago
4 ☐ 6-9 years ago
5 ☐ I0 years ago or more
9 ☐ Don't know

9a. Have you seen a doctor or anyone else about the chest or lung conditions you mentioned previously? | 9a. | (101) 1 ☐ Yes — Ask b
2 ☐ No — SKIP to 10

b. What is the name of the doctor you see?

_____

c. What type of doctor is he? c. (102) 1 ☐ General Practitioner
2 ☐ Internist
3 ☐ Osteopath
4 ☐ Surgeon
5 ☐ Lung specialist
6 ☐ Allergist
7 ☐ Other — Specify - - - . - - - - . - - - -

d, Who initially referred you to this doctor? d. (103) 1 ☐ No one
2 ☐ He's the regular doctor
3 ☐ Another physician
4 ☐ Health nurse
5 ☐ Clinic
6 ☐ Family
7 ☐ Other — Specify _____

9e. How long after you first developed the problem did you see him?   **9e.**

(104)
1 ☐ 1-6 days
2 ☐ 1-7 weeks
3 ☐ 2-6 months
4 ☐ 7-11 months
5 ☐ One year or more
9 ☐ Don't know

f. What did he say the condition or conditions affecting your chest were?   **f.**

_____

_____

_____

_____

_____

DATA PREPARATION USE ONLY		
(105) 1 ☐	(110) 1 ☐	(115) 1 ☐
(106) 1 ☐	(111) 'cl	
(107) ' c 1	(112) 1 ☐	
(108) ' c 1	(113) 1 ☐	
(109) 1 cl	(114) 1 ☐	

g. When you see the doctor about your chest condition, how often do you receive a chest x-ray?   **g.**

(116)
1 ☐ At every visit
2 ☐ At every other visit
3 ☐ Less often than every other visit

h. Does he prescribe the medicine for the condition?   **ho**

(117)
1 ☐ ＊▥＊ – ▥＊& i
2 ☐ No – *SKIP* to j

i. How is the medicine taken?   **i.**

	Yes	No
Swallowed . . . . (118)	1 ☐	2 ☐
Breathed . . . . (119)	1 ☐	2 ☐
Injected . . . . (120)	1 ☐	2 ☐
Other – Specify_____ (121)	1 ☐	2 ☐

j. Has he told you to do any of these other things for it?   **j.**

	Yes	No
Breathing exercises. . . . . (122)	1 ☐	2 ☐
Use a breathing machine . . . . (123)	1 ☐	2 ☐
Stop smoking . . . . (124)	1 ☐	2 ☐
Decrease smoking . . . . (125)	1 ☐	2 ☐
Regular checkup. . . . . (126)	1 ☐	2 ☐
Lots of rest . . . . (127)	1 ☐	2 ☐
Decrease activity . . . . (128)	. . .	2 ☐
Other – *Specify*_____ (129)	1 ☐	2 ☐

k. When was the last time you saw him?   **k.**

(130)
1 ☐ Less than 1 month ago
2 ☐ 1-3 months ago
3 ☐ 4–6 months ago
4 ☐ 7-11 months ago
5 ☐ 1 year ago or more
9 ☐ Don't know

9l. Where do you usually see him?	9l.	(131)	1 ☐ At his office 2 ☐ At a clinic 3 ☐ At home 4 ☐ Other — Specify _____	
m. How long will it be until your next appointment?	m.	(132)	1 ☐ Less than I month 2 ☐ I-3 months 3 ☐ 4-6 months 4 ☐ 7-I I months 5 ☐ I year or more 9 ☐ Don't know	
10. Within the past 12 months, has your chest condition gotten worse, gotten better, or stayed about the same?	10.	(133)	1 ☐ Gotten worse 2 ☐ Gotten better 3 ☐ Stayed about the same	
11. Have you ever been disabled because of any chest condition?	11.	(134)	1 ☐ Yes 2 ☐ No	
12. Have you ever stayed overnight in a hospital because of a chest condition?	12.	(135)	1 ☐ Yes 2 ☐ No	
13. What was your job status one month before you first had a problem with a chest or lung condition?	13.	(136)	1 ☐ Retired because of age 2 ☐ Retired because of disability 3 ☐ Unemployed 4 ☐ Working ful I-time 5 ☐ Working part-time 6 ☐ Housewife with full duties 7 ☐ Housewife with partial or no duties 8 ☐ Other — Specify _____	
14a. As a result of your chest or lung condition, has there been a change in your job status?	14a.	(137)	1 ☐ Yes — Ask b 2 ☐ No — SKIP to IS	
b. What is it now?	b.	(138)	1 ☐ Retired because of di sabi l i ty 2 ☐ Unemployed 3 ☐ Working only part-time 4 ☐ Changed to easier job 5 ☐ Housewife with partial duties 6 ☐ Housewife with no duties 7 ☐ Other — Specify _____	
15. How many work days would you estimate you have lost during the past 12 months because of your chest or lung condition, excluding colds or flu?	15.	(139)	1 ☐ None 2 ☐ I-4 days 3 ☐ 5-9 days 4 ☐ IO-14 days 5 ☐ I5—I9 days 6 ☐ 20-29 days 7 ☐ 30 days or more	

H. Supplement C—Cardiovascular

HSM-411-4 (PAGE 1)
REV. 5/71

Form Approved
O.M. B. No. 68-R 1 184

DEPARTMENT OF HEALTH, EDUCATION, AND WELFARE
PUBLIC HEALTH SERVICE
HEALTH SERVICES AND MENTAL HEALTH ADMINISTRATION
NATIONAL CENTER FOR HEALTH STATISTICS
HEALTH AND NUTRITION EXAMINATION SURVEY

SUPPLEMENT C – CARDIOVASCULAR

a. Name (Last, first, middle)

b. Deck No. **141**

c. Sample No. ___ ___

READ – Earlier you mentioned having a history of either chest pains, chest discomfort or heaviness, leg pains while walking, or heart failure. Here are some additional questions about it.

Ia. Was the problem that of chest pains, chest discomfort, pressure, or heaviness?

Ia. (001) 1 ☐ Yes – Ask b
2 ☐ No – SKIP to 2a

b. How would you best describe this pain or discomfort?

b.

	Yes	No
H e a v i n e s s.,...................... (002)	1 ☐	2 ☐
Burning sensation.................... (003)	1 ☐	2 ☐
Tightness,....................... (004)	1 ☐	2 ☐
Stabbing pain..................... (005)	1 ☐	2 ☐
Pressure.. .... (006)	1 ☐	2 ☐
Sharp pain . . . . . , ... , ... (007)	1 ☐	2 ☐
Shooting pains .... (008)	1 ☐	2 ☐

c. Have you had it more than THREE times?

c. (009) 1 ☐ Yes
2 ☐ No

d. Have you been bothered by this within the past 12 months?

d. (010) 1 ☐ Yes
2 ☐ No

e. How old were you when you first had it?

e. (011) 1 ☐ 10 – 19 years old
2 ☐ 20 – 29 years old
3 ☐ 30 – 39 years old
4 ☐ 40 – 49 years old
5 ☐ 50 – 59 years old
6 ☐ 60 years old or older

f. Do you get it if you walk at an ordinary pace on level ground?

f. (012) 1 ☐ Yes
2 ☐ No

g. Do you get it if you walk uphill or hurry?

g. (013) 1 ☐ Yes – Ask h
2 ☐ No – SKIP ◆☐ k

1h. What do you do if you get it while walking?	1h.		Yes	No
stop.		(014)	1 ☐	2 ☐
Slow down		(0)5	'ol	2 ☐
Continue at same pace.		016	1 ☐	2 ☐
Take medicine.		(017)	1 ☐	2 ☐

i. If you do stop or slow down, is it relieved or not?	i.	(018)	1 ☐ Relieved – Ask j
			2 ☐ Not relieved – SKIP to k

j. How soon?	j.	(0)9	1 ☐ Less than 10 minutes
			2 ☐ 10 minutes or more

k. When you get pain or discomfort, where is it located?	k.		Yes	No
Upper middle chest , ...		(020)	1 ☐	2 ☐
Lower middle chest.		(021)	1 ☐	2 ☐
Left side of chest.		(022)	1 ☐	2 ☐
Left arm		(023)	c ☐	2 ☐
Right side of chest		(024)	c ☐	2 ☐
Other – Specify ———————		025	1 ☐	2 ☐

l. Do any of these things tend to bring it on?	l.		Yes	No
Excitement or emotion		(026)	1 ☐	2 ☐
Stooping over		(027)	1 ☐	2 ☐
Eating a heavy meal		(028)	1 ☐	2 ☐
Coughing spells		(029)	1 ☐	2 ☐
Cold wind		(030)	1 ☐	2 ☐
Exertion		(031)	1 ☐	2 ☐

2a. Have you ever had severe pain across the front of your chest lasting for half an hour or more?	2a.	(032)	1 ☐ Yes – Ask b
			2 ☐ No – SKIP to 3a

b. How many of these attacks have you had?	b.	(033)	1 ☐ One
			2 ☐ 2 – 3
			3 ☐ 4 or more

c. What was the date of your last attack?	c.	(034)	Month	Year
			— —	— —

d. What was the duration of the pain during your last attack?	d.	(035)	1 ☐ 30 – 59 minutes
			2 ☐ – 2 hours
			3 ☐ 3 – 5 hours
			4 ☐ 6 – 11 hours
			5 ☐ 12 – 23 hours
			6 ☐ 24 – 47 hours
			7 ☐ 2 days or more

2e. Did you see a doctor about this lost attack?	2e.	(036) 1 ☐ **Yes** – Ask f 2 ☐ No – SKIP to 3a
f. What did he say it was? _____ _____ _____ _____	f.	DATA **PREPARATION** USE ONLY (037) 1 ☐ 041 1 ☐ (038) 1 ☐ 042 1 ☐ (039) 1 ☐ 043 1 ☐ (040) 1 ☐ 044 1 ☐
3a. Do you get pain or discomfort in either leg while walking?	3a.	(045) 1 ☐ Yes – Ask b 2 ☐ No – SKIP to 4a
b. Do you also get this pain in your legs while standing still?	b.	(046) 1 ☐ Yes 2 ☐ No
c. In what parts of your leg do you feel this pain?	c.	(047) 1 ☐ Lower part (calf) 2 ☐ Upper part (thigh) 3 ☐ Both lower and upper parts
d. Do you get the pain in your legs while quiet or while sitting?	d.	(048) 1 ☐ Yes 2 ☐ No
e. Do you get it when you walk up a hill in a hurry?	e.	(049) 1 ☐ Yes 2 ☐ No
f. Do you get it when you walk at an ordinary pace on level ground?	f.	(050) 1 ☐ Yes 2 ☐ No
g. Does the pain in your legs come on after you have taken a few steps?	g.	(051) 1 ☐ Yes 2 ☐ No
h. Does the pain disappear while you ore still walking?	h.	(052) 1 ☐ Yes 2 ☐ ho
i. What do you do when you get it while you are walking? stop. . . . . Slow down . . . . Continue at same pace. . . . . Take medicine. . . . . , . . , . .	i.	Yes No (053) 1 ☐ 2 ☐ (054) 1 ☐ 2 ☐ (055) 1 ☐ 2 ☐ (056) 1 ☐ 2 ☐
j. If you stop, is it relieved or not?	j.	(057) 1 [I] Relieved – Ask k 2 ☐ Not relieved – SKIP to l
k. How soon after stopping?	k.	(058) 1 ☐ Less than IO minutes 2 ☐ IO minutes or more
l. Is the pain more likely to occur when you are hurrying than when you are walking at a slower, more even pace?	l.	(059) 1 ☐ Yes 2 ☐ No

4a. Have you ever seen a doctor about chest pains, chest discomfort, pains in the legs while walking, or heart failure?

b. What is the name of the doctor?

_____

c. What type of doctor is he?

d. Who initially referred you to this doctor?

No one. . . . .

He's the regular doctor . . . .

Another doctor . . . .

Family.. . . . .

Clinic.. . . . .

Health nurse . . . .

Other – Specify _____

e. How long after this trouble first started did you first visit your doctor about it?

f. At that time, what did he say the problem was?

_____

_____

g. Did you have a cardiogram at the first visit?

h. Did you have one at a later visit?

i. How long was it from the time of the first visit?

4a.	(060) 1 ☐ Yes – Ask b
	☐ ☐ – *SKIP* ◀☐ 5
c.	(061) 1 ☐ General practitioner
	2 ☐ Osteopath
	3 ☐ Heart specialist
	4 ☐ Other specialist
	5 ☐ Other – Specify _____
	9 ☐ Don't know

d.

	Yes	No
(062)	1 ☐	2 ☐
(063)	1 ☐	2 ☐
(064)	1 ☐	2 ☐
(065)	1 ☐	2 ☐
(066)	1 ☐	2 ☐
(067)	1 ☐	2 ☐
(068)	1 ☐	2 ☐

e. (069)
1 ☐ Less than I day
2 ☐ I – 2 days
3 ☐ 3 – 6 days
4 ☐ I – 3 weeks
5 ☐ I – 5 months
6 ☐ 6 – I I months
7 ☐ I year or more
9 ☐ Don't remember

g. (070)
1 ☐ Yes
2 ☐ No

h. (071)
1 ☐ Yes – Ask i
2 ☐ No – *SKIP* to 4j

i. (072)
1 ☐ I – 2 days
2 ☐ 3 – 6 days
3 ☐ I – 3 weeks
4 ☐ I – 5 months
5 ☐ 6 – I I months
6 ☐ I year or more
9 ☐ Don't know

4j. Did you have a chest X-ray at the first visit? 4j. (073) 1 ☐ Yes
                                                       2 ☐ No

k. Did you have one at a later visit? k. (074) 1 ☐ Yes — *Ask* l
                                                       2 ☐ No — *SKIP* to m

l. How long was it from the time of the first visit? l. (075) 1 ☐ 1 — 2 days
                                                       2 ☐ 3 — 6 days
                                                       3 ☐ 1 — 3 weeks
                                                       4 ☐ 1 — 5 months
                                                       5 ☐ 6 — 11 months
                                                       6 ☐ 1 year or more
                                                       9 ☐ Don't know

m. Have you had any other tests for this condition? (such as blood or urine) m. (076) 1 ☐ Yes
                                                       2 ☐ No

n. Did the doctor prescribe medicines to take for your condition? n. (077) 1 ☐ Yes — *Ask* o
                                                       2 ☐ No — *SKIP* to p

o. How do you take the medicine? o.

	Yes	No
Swallowed . . . . (078)	1 ☐	2 ☐
Under the tongue . . . . (079)	1 ☐	2 ☐
Injected . . . . (080)	1 ☐	2 ☐
Other — Specify _____ (081)	1 ☐	2 ☐

p. Has he told you to do any of these other things? p.

	Yes	No
Make regular visits . . . . (082)	1 ☐	2 ☐
Have regular cardiograms . . . . (083)	1 ☐	2 ☐
Decrease activity . . . . (084)	1 ☐	2 ☐
Increase activity . . . . (085)	1 ☐	2 ☐
Rest . . . . (086)	1 ☐	2 ☐
Do exercises . . . . (087)	1 ☐	2 ☐
Stop smoking . . . . (088)	1 ☐	2 ☐
Other — Specify _____ (089)	1 ☐	2 ☐

q. When was the last time you saw him? q. (090) 1 ☐ Less than 1 month ago
                                                       2 ☐ 1 — 3 months ago
                                                       3 ☐ 4 — 6 months ago
                                                       4 ☐ 7 — 11 months ago
                                                       5 ☐ 1 year ago or more
                                                       9 ☐ Don't remember

r. Where do you usually see him? r. (091) 1 ☐ At his office
                                                       2 ☐ At a clinic
                                                       3 ☐ At home
                                                       4 ☐ Other — Specify _____

4s. **How** long will it be until your next visit?	4s. (092)	1 ☐ Less than I month 2 ☐ I – 3 months 3 ☐ 4 – 6 months 4 ☐ 7 – I I months 5 ☐ I year or more 9 ☐ Don't know
t. Would you say that the treatments you have had have done you any good?	t. (093)	1 ☐ No, not at all 2 ☐ Yes, partly 3 ☐ Yes, quite a bit
5. Within the past 12 months, would you say that your condition has gotten worse, gotten better, or stayed about the same?	5. (094)	1 ☐ Gotten worse 2 ☐ Gotten better 3 ☐ Stayed about the same
6. Have you ever been disabled because of chest pain, leg pain, or heart failure?	6. (095)	1 ☐ Yes 2 ☐ ✂☐
7. Have you ever stayed overnight in a hospital because of chest pain, leg pain, or heart failure?	7. (096)	1 ☐ Yes 2 ☐ No
8. What was your job status one month before you first developed chest pain, leg pain, or heart fai l ure?	8. (097)	1 ☐ Retired because of **age** 2 ☐ Reti red because of di sabi li ty 3 ☐ Unemployed 4 ☐ Working full-time 5 ☐ Working part-time 6 ☐ Housewife with ful l duties 7 ☐ Housewife with partial or no duties 8 ☐ Other – Specify _____ _____
9a. As a result of your condition, has there been a change in your job status?	9a. (098)	1 ☐ Yes – Ask b 2 ☐ No – SKIP to 10
b. What is it now?	b. (099)	1 ☐ Retired because of disabi li ty 2 ☐ Unemployed 3 ☐ Working only part-time 4 ☐ Changed to easier job 5 ☐ Housewife with partial duties 6 ☐ Housewife with no duties 7 ☐ Other – Specify _____ _____
10. How many work days would you estimate you have lost during the past 12 months because of your heart condition?	10. (100)	1 ☐ None 2 ☐ I – 4 days 3 ☐ 5 – 9 days 4 ☐ IO – I4 days 5 ☐ I5 – I9 days 6 ☐ 20 – 29 days 7 ☐ 30 days or more

J. Body Measurements

(R/\ 1 2.7A (Formerly HSM-425-7A)
\-74

Form Approved
O.M.B. No. 68-R1184

DEPARTMENT OF HEALTH, EDUCATION, AND WELFARE

PUBLIC HEALTH SERVICE
HEALTH RESOURCES ADMINISTRATION
NATIONAL CENTER FOR HEALTH STATISTICS

HEALTH EXAMINATION SURVEY

BODY MEASUREMENTS

a. Deck No.	**b.** Examiner No.	**c.** Recorder No.
111	__ __	

NOTE Measuremknt in cm. unless otherwise specified.

Measure left side also if the last digit of examinee's sample number is 3 or 6.

1. Bitrochanteric breadth   1.   (009) __ __ . __

2. Elbow breadth   2.   (001) RIGHT SIDE __ __ . __   (002) LEFT SIDE __ __ . __

3. Upper arm girth   3.   (003) RIGHT SIDE __ __ . __   (004) LEFT SIDE __ __ . __

Chest circumference
4a. Full expiration   4a.   (018) __ __ __ . __

 b. Full inspiration   b.   (017) __ __ __ . __

5. Triceps skinfold (mm.)   5.   (005) RIGHT SIDE __ __ . __   (006) LEFT SIDE __ __ . __

6. Subscapular skinfold (mm.)   6.   (007) RIGHT SIDE __ __ . __   (0008) LEFT SIDE __ __ . __

7. Sitting height   7.   (010) __ __ . __

When both sides ore measured
8. Is examinee right or left handed?   8.   (016)
☐ Right handed
2 ☐ Left handed
3 ☐ Uses both hands about the same
4 ☐ Not sure
8 ☐ Not applicable

9. Weight (lbs.)   9.   (013) __ __ __ . __

10a. Standing height (cm.)   10a.   (014) __ __ __ . __

 b. Standing height (inches)   b.   __ __ __ /

NOTES

Sample Number
N⁰ 98743

K. General Medical Examination

HRA-12-3
FORMERLY HSM-425-3
(7/74)

DEPARTMENT OF HEALTH, EDUCATION, AND WELFARE
PUBLIC HEALTH SERVICE
HEALTH RESOURCES ADMINISTRATION
NATIONAL CENTER FOR HEALTH STATISTICS

GENERAL MEDICAL EXAMINATION – AGES 25–74

HEALTH EXAMINATION SURVEY

Form Approved
O.M.B. No. 68-R1184

ASSURANCE OF CONFIDENTIALITY
All information which would permit identification of the individual will be held strictly confidential, will be used only by persons engaged in and for the purposes of the survey, and will not be disclosed or released to others for any other purposes (22 FR 1687).

a. Name (Last, first, middle)	**b.** Deck No.	**c.** Pulse	**d.** Blood pressure
	231	(001) _ _ _	Systolic (002) _ _ _ Diastolic (003) _ _ _

1. HEAD, EYES, EARS, NOSE, AND THROAT:

(004) 1 ☐ Findings
2 ☐ No findings

If findings, *mark* applicable box and *continue* with a.
If no findings, SKIP to 2a.

Yes

a. Conjunctival injection . . . . . . (010) 1 ☐

b. Fi li form papi l lary atrophy of tongue . . . . (019) 1 ☐

c. Fungi form papi l l ary hypertrophy of tongue . . . . (020) 1 ☐

d. Fissures of tongue . . . . (022) 1 ☐

e. Serrations or swelling of tongue (023) 1 ☐

f. Scarlet beefy tongue . . . . (024) 1 ☐

g. Other – Specify _____

_____ (029) 1 ☐

2a. THYROID EVALUATION:
(WHO Classification)

(030) 1 ☐ Group 0
2 ☐ Group I
3 ☐ Group 2
4 ☐ Group 3

b. OTHER THYROID FINDINGS:

(031) 1 ☐ Findings
2 ☐ No findings (GO to 3)

R L Both

(1) Tenderness. . . . . (032) 1 ☐ 2 ☐ 3 ☐

(2) Nodule. . . . . (033) 1 ☐ 2 ☐ 3 ☐

(3) Isthmus . . . . (034) 1 ☐

(4) Other – Describe _____

_____ (035) 1 ☐

3. CARDIOVASCULAR EVALUATIONS:

(043) 1 ☐ Findings
2 ☐ No findings

If findings, *applicable* box and continue with a.
If no findings, SKIP to 4.

Yes

a. Cyanosis . . . . (044) 1 ☐

b. Irregular pulse. . . . . (045) 1 ☐

4. ABDOMINAL EVALUATION:

(048) 1 ☐ Findings
2 ☐ No findings

If findings, mark applicable box and continue with a.
If no findings, SKIP to 5.

Yes

a. Hepatomegaly. . . . . (049) 1 ☐

b. Splenomegaly . . . . (050) 1 ☐

c. Uterine enlargement . . . . (051) 1 ☐

d. Umbilical hernia. . . . . (052) 1 ☐

e. Mass(es). . . . . (054) 1 ☐

(1) Area(s) – Enter number(s) (055) _ _ _ _ _

(2) Other findings – Describe (056) 1 ☐

_____

f. Surgical scars . . . . (057) 1 ☐

(1) Area(s) – Enter number(s) (058) _ _ _ _ _

(2) Other findings – Describe (059) 1 ☐

_____

S A M P L E

N 98743

5. MUSCUCOSKELETAL EVALUATION:

If findings, murk applicable box and describe.
If no findings, SKIP to 6.

Findings – Describe ↗

_____

_____

(062) 1 ☐   Findings

2 ☐ **No** findings

Yes

(066) 1 ☐

---

6. NEUROLOGICAL EVALUATION:

If findings, mark applicable box ond continue with a.
If no findings, SKIP to 7.

a.   Absent knee jerks . . . .

b. Absent ankle jerks . . . .

c. Other findings – Describe ↗

_____

_____

(067) 1 ☐   Findings

2 ☐ **No** findings

Yes

(068) 1 ☐

(069) 1 ☐

(073) 1 ☐

---

7. SKIN EVALUATION:

If findings, mark applicable box and continue with a.
If no findings, SKIP to 8.

a. Petechiae – Describe ↗

_____

_____

b. Ecchymoses – Describe ↗

_____

_____

c. Other findings – Describe₃

_____

(074) 1 ☐ Findings

2 ☐ No findings

Yes

(079) 1 ☐

(082) 1 ☐

(083) 1 ☐

8a. Obesity . . . .

b. No obesity . . . .

(093) 1 ☐

2 ☐

---

9. Name of physician

Comments

SAMPLE NUMBER

N₂   98743

80

DEPARTMENT OF HEALTH, EDUCATION, AND WELFARE

PUBLIC HEALTH SERVICE
HEALTH RESOURCES ADMINISTRATION
NATIONAL CENTER FOR HEALTH STATISTICS

HEALTH EXAMINATION SURVEY

GENERAL MEDICAL EXAMINATION

Form Approved
O.M.B. No. 68-RI 184

ASSURANCE OF CONFIDENTIALITY
All information which would permit identification of the individual will be held strictly confidential, will be used only by persons engaged in and for the purposes of the survey, and will not be disclosed or released to others for any other purposes (22 FR 1687).

Deck No. 232

A. EXTERNAL EAR (Except canal)

	Right	Left
1. No findings – SKIP to B	(001) 1 ☐	(002) 1 ☐
2. Findings – Continue with 3 . . 2.	2 ☐	2 ☐
3. Operative scar . . . 3.	(003) 1 ☐	(004) 1 ☐
4. Other – Describe . 4.	(005) 1 ☐	(006) 1 ☐
5. Pierced ears . . . . 5.	(007) 1 ☐ Yes	2 ☐ No

B. AUDITORY CANAL

	Right	Left
1. No findings – SKIP to C . . . . . 1.	(008) 1 ☐	(009) 1 ☐
2. Findings – Continue with 3 . . 2.	2 ☐	2 ☐
3. Occluded: a. Partially . . . . . 3a.	(010) 1 ☐	(011) 1 ☐
b. Completely . . . . b.	2 ☐	2 ☐
4. Occluded by: a. Cerumen . . . . . 4a.	(012) 1 ☐	(013) 1 ☐
b. Other – Describe b.	2 ☐	2 ☐

C. DRUM

	Right	Left
1. No findings – SKIP to D . . . . . . 1.	(014) 1 ☐	(015) 1 ☐
2. Findings – Continue with 4 . . . 2.	2 ☐	2 ☐
3. Not visible . . . . . 3.	3 ☐	3 ☐
4. Dull (Opaque) . . . . 4.	(016) 1 ☐	(017) 1 ☐
5. Transparent . . . . . 5.	2 ☐	2 ☐
6. Bulging . . . . . . 6.	(018) 1 ☐	(019) 1 ☐ cl
7. Retracted . . . . . 7.	2 ☐	2 ☐
8. Calcium plaques . . 8.	(020) 1 ☐	(021) 1 ☐
9. Other findings – Describe . . . . . . 9.	(022) 1 ☐	(023) 1 ☐

C. DRUM – Continued

	Right	Left
10. Red . . . . .10.	(024) 1 ☐	(025) 1 ☐
11. Other discolorations 11.	2 ☐	2 ☐
12. Fluid . . . . . . .12.	(026) 1 ☐	(027) 1 ☐
13. Scars . . . . .13.	(028) 1 ☐	(029) 1 ☐
14. Perforated a. With discharge 14a.	(030) 030 1 ☐	(031) 031 1 ☐
b. Without discharge . b.	2 ☐	2 ☐

D. NARES

	Right	Left
1. No findings – SKIP to E . . . . . . 1.	(032) 1 ☐	(033) 1 ☐
2. Findings – Continue with 3 . . 2.	2 ☐	2 ☐
3. Obstruction a. Acute . . . . 3a.	(034) 1 ☐	(035) 1 ☐
b. Chronic . . . . . b.	2 ☐	2 ☐
4. Other significant findings – a. Deviated septum . 4a.	(036) 1 ☐	(037) 1 ☐
b. Swollen turbinates b.	(038) 1 ☐	(039) 1 ☐
c. Chronic inflammation c.	(040) 1 ☐	(041) 1 ☐
d. Other -Describe . d .	(042) 1 ☐	(043) 1 ☐

E. NECK

	Right	Left
1. No findings – SKIP to F . . . . . . 1.	(044) 1 ☐	
2. Findings – Continue with 3 . . 2.	2 ☐	
3. Adenopathy . . . . . 3.	(045) 1 ☐	
4. Tracheal deviation. 4.	(046) 1 ☐	
5. Other – Describe . . 5.	(047) 1 ☐	

Sample Number

N⁰ 98743

F. CHEST

1. Auscultation

(048) 1 ☐ No findings — SKIP to G

2 ☐ Findings

		Dimin. brth. sounds	Absent b.s.	Bronchial b.s.	Rales	Rhonchi	Wheeze
Right chest Upper lobe		(049) 1 ☐	2 ☐	(050) 1 ☐	(051) 1 ☐	(052) 1 ☐	(053) 1 ☐
Middle lobe		(054) 1 ☐	2 ☐	(055) 1 ☐	(056) 1 ☐	(057) 1 ☐	(058) 1 ☐
Lower lobe		(059) 1 ☐	2 ☐	(060) 1 ☐	(061) 1 ☐	(062) 1 ☐	(063) 1 ☐
Left chest Upper lobe		(064) 1 ☐	2 ☐	(065) 1 ☐	(066) 1 ☐	(067) 1 ☐	(068) 1 ☐
Lower lobe		(069) 1 ☐	2 ☐	(070) 1 ☐	(071) 1 ☐	(072) 1 ☐	(073) 1 ☐

2. Other chest findings

(074) 1 ☐ None   2 ☐ Findings _____

G. HEART

1. P.M.I. . . . . 1.   (075) 1 ☐ Felt   2 ☐ Not felt

2. Interspace . . . . 2.   (076) 4 ☐ 5 ☐ 6 ☐ 7 ☐

3. Midclavicular line . . . . 3.   (077) 1 ☐ At   2 ☐ Inside   3 ☐ Outside

4. Thrills . . . . 4.   (078) 1 ☐ Absent   2 ☐ Present

   a. Systolic. . . . . a.   (079) 1 ☐ Base   2 ☐ Apex

   b. Diastolic . . . . b.   (080) 1 ☐ Base   2 ☐ Apex

5. Heart sounds

   a. 1st heart sound . . . . 5a.   (081) 1 ☐ Normal   2 ☐ Accentuated   3 ☐ Diminished

   b. 2nd heart sound . . . . b.   (082) 1 ☐ Normal   2 ☐ Accentuated   3 ☐ Diminished

6. Murmurs . . . . 6.   (083) 1 ☐ None — Skip to 7

MURMUR(S)

	SYSTOLIC MURMUR(S)	DIASTOLIC MURMUR(S)
a. Type. . . . . a.	(084) 1 ☐ Functional 2 ☐ Organic 9 ☐ Don't know	(085) 1 ☐ Functional 2 ☐ Organic 9 ☐ Don't know

   b. Location

	GRADE	GRADE
(1) Apex . . . . b(1)	(086) 1☐ 2☐ 3☐ 4☐ 5☐ 6☐	(087) 1☐ 2☐ 3☐ 4☐ 5☐ 6☐
(2) Midprecordium . . . . (2)	(088) 1☐ 2☐ 3☐ 4☐ 5☐ 6☐	(089) 1☐ 2☐ 3☐ 4☐ 5☐ 6☐
(3) Left base. . . . . (3)	(090) 1☐ 2☐ 3☐ 4☐ 5☐ 6☐	(091) 1☐ 2☐ 3☐ 4☐ 5☐ 6☐
(4) Right base . . . . (4)	(092) 1☐ 2☐ 3☐ 4☐ 5☐ 6☐	(093) 1☐ 2☐ 3☐ 4☐ 5☐ 6☐

Continue with 6c, "Origin" on Page 3

Sample Number

Nº 98743

82

G. HEART — Continued
6. Murmurs — Continued
c. Origin

		Systolic	Diastolic	Both
(1) Mitral	6c.(1)	(094) 1 ☐	2 ☐	3 ☐
(2) Aortic.	(2)	(095) 1 ☐	2 ☐	3 ☐
(3) Tricuspid.	(3)	096 1 ☐	2 ☐	3 ☐
(4) Pulmonic	(4)	097 1 ☐	2 ☐	3 ☐
(5) ASD : : : : : : : : : : : : : : :	(5)	(098) 1 ☐	2 ☐	3 ☐
(6) VSD : :	(6)	(099) 9 1 ☐	2 ☐	3 ☐
(7) Other	(7)	(100) 1 ☐	2 ☐	3 ☐
(8) Don't know	(8)	(101) 9 E1		

7. Other cardiac or cardiovascular findings

102 1 ☐ No — Skip to *H*   2 ☐ **Yes** — Continue with *7a*

a. Edema . . . . **7a.**   103 1 ☐

b. Other — Describe . . . . b.   (104) 1 ☐

_____

_____

c. Neck vein distension . . . . c.   105 1 ☐

H. PULSE — ARTERIAL EVALUATION
1. Palpation

		Normal	Sclerotic	Tortuous	Sclerotic and Tortuous
a. Right radial	1a.	106 1 ☐	2 ☐	3 ☐	4 ☐
b. Right femoral	b.	(107) 1 ☐	2 ☐	3 ☐	4 ☐
c. Right dorsalis pedis	c.	108 1 ☐	2 ☐	3 ☐	4 ☐
d. Left radial	d.	(109) 1 ☐	2 ☐	3 ☐	4 ☐
e. Left femoral	e.	(110) 1 ☐	2 ☐	3 ☐	4 ☐
f. Left dorsalis pedis	f.	(111) 1 ☐	2 ☐	3 ☐	4 ☐

2. Pulsations

		Normal	Diminished	Bounding	Absent
a. Right radial	2a.	112 1 ☐	2 ☐	3 ☐	4 ☐
b. Right femoral	b.	(113) 1 ☐	2 ☐	3 ☐	4 ☐
c. Right dorsalis pedis	c.	114 1 ☐	2 ☐	3 ☐	4 ☐
d. Other — Describe	d.	115 1 c1	2 ☐	3 ☐	4 ☐

_____

_____

		Normal	Diminished	Bounding	Absent
e. Left radial	e.	116 1 ☐	2 ☐	3 ☐	4 ☐
f. Left femoral	f.	8 117 1 ☐	2 ☐	3 ☐	4 ☐
g. Left dorsalis pedis	g.	(118) 1 ☐	2 ☐	3 ☐	4 ☐
h. Other — Describe	h.	(119) 1 ☐	2 ☐	3 ☐	4 ☐

_____

_____

Sample Number

N⁰ 98743

I. KNEES

(120) 1 ☐ Findings — Continue with 1
2 ☐ No findings — Skip to J

1. Bony irregularity

		R	L	Both
a. Genu varum	lo. (121)	1 ☐	2 ☐	3 ☐
b. Genu valgum	b. (122)	1 ☐	2 ☐	3 ☐
c. Genu recurvatum	c. (123)	1 ☐	2 ☐	3 ☐
d. Fixed flexion	d. (124)	1 ☐	2 ☐	3 ☐
e. Other — Describe	e. (125)	1 ☐	2 ☐	3 ☐

_____

2. Pain on motion

		Act.	Pas.	Both	Tenderness	
a. Right medial	2a. (126)	1 ☐	2 ☐	3 ☐	(127)	1 ☐
b. Right lateral	b. (128)	1 ☐	2 ☐	3 ☐	(129)	1 ☐
c. Right diffuse	c. (130)	1 ☐	2 ☐	3 ☐	(131)	1 ☐
d. Left medial	d. (132)	1 ☐	2 ☐	3 ☐	133	1 ☐
e. Left lateral	e. (134)	1 ☐	2 ☐	3 ☐	(135)	1 ☐
f. Left diffuse	f. (136)	1 cl	2 ☐	3 ☐	(137)	1 ☐
g. Right suprapatellar	g.				(138)	1 ☐
h. Left suprapatellar	h.				139	1 ☐
i. Right infrapatellar	i.				(140)	1 ☐
j. Left infrapatellar	j.				(141)	1 cl

3. Other findings

		R	L	Both
a. Swelling	3a. (142)	1 ☐	2 ☐	3 ☐
b. Fluid	b. (143)	1 ☐	2 ☐	3 ☐
c. Soft tissue proliferation	c. (144)	1 ☐	2 ☐	3 ☐
d. Subpatellar crepitus	d. (145)	1 C l	2 ☐	3 ☐
e. Muscular wasting thigh	e. (146)	1 Cl	2 ☐	3 ☐
f. Other — Describe	f. (147)	1 ☐	2 ☐	3 ☐

_____

J. HIPS

(148) 1 ☐ Findings — Continue with 1
2 ☐ No findings — Skip to K

1. Pain on motion

		ACTIVE			PASSIVE		
		R	L	Both	R	L	Both
a. Extension	lo. (149)	1 ☐	2 ☐	3 ☐	(150) 1 ☐	2 ☐	3 ☐
b. Flexion	b. (151)	1 ☐	2 ☐	3 ☐	(152) 1 ☐	2 ☐	3 ☐
c. Abduction	c. (153)	1 ☐	2 ☐	3 ☐	(154) 1 ☐	2 ☐	3 ☐
d. Adduction	d. (155)	1 ☐	2 ☐	3 ☐	(156) 1 ☐	2 ☐	3 ☐
e. Ext. rot.	e. (157)	1 ☐	2 ☐	3 ☐	(158) 1 ☐	2 ☐	3 ☐
f. Int. rot	f. (159)	1 ☐	2 ☐	3 ☐	(160) 1 ☐	2 ☐	3 ☐

Sample Number

N? 98743

J. HIPS — Continued

1. Other findings

	R	L	Both
a. Muscle wasting (glutea) . . . . . 1a.	(161) 1	2	3
b. Trochanter tenderness. . . . . b.	(162) 1	2	3
c. Groin tenderness . . . . . c.	(163) 1	2	3
d. Other — Describe —	(164) 1	2	3

K. JOINTS

(165) 1 ☐ No findings — Skip to L
2 ☐ Findings — Describe and continue with 1

MANIFESTATIONS

Other joints	Tender	Swelling	Deformity	Limitation	Heberden's nodes	Pain on motion	Other
1. Shoulder	(166) 1☐R 3☐B 2☐L	(167) 1☐R 3☐B 2☐L	(168) 1☐R 3☐B 2☐L	(169) 1☐R 3☐B 2☐L		(170) 1☐R 3☐B 2☐L	(171) 1☐R 3☐B 2☐L
2. Elbow	(172) 1☐R 3☐B 2☐L	(173) 1☐R 3☐B 2☐L	(174) 1☐R 3☐B 2☐L	(175) 1☐R 3☐B 2☐L		(176) 1☐R 3☐B 2☐L	(177) 1☐R 3☐B 2☐L
3. Wrist	(178) 1☐R 3☐B 2☐L	(179) 1☐R 3☐B 2☐L	(180) 1☐R 3☐B 2☐L	(181) 1☐R 3☐B 2☐L		(182) 1☐R 3☐B 2☐L	(183) 1☐R 3☐B 2☐L

	RIGHT / LEFT	RIGHT / LEFT	RIGHT / LEFT	RIGHT / LEFT	RIGHT / LEFT	RIGHT / LEFT	RIGHT / LEFT
4. Metacarpo-phalangeal (No. involved)	(184) 1 2 3 4 5 / (185)	(186) 1 2 3 4 5 / (187)	(188) 1 2 3 4 5 / (189)	(190) 1 2 3 4 5 / (191)		(192) 1 2 3 4 5 / (193)	(194) 1 2 3 4 5 / (195)
5. Proximal-inter-phalangeal (No. involved)	(196) 1 2 3 4 5 / (197)	(198) 1 2 3 4 5 / (199)	(200) 1 2 3 4 5 / (201)	(202) 1 2 3 4 5 / (203)		(204) 1 2 3 4 5 / (205)	(206) 1 2 3 4 5 / (207)
6. Distal-inter-phalangeal (No. involved)	(208) 1 2 3 4 5 / (209)	(210) 1 2 3 4 5 / (211)	(212) 1 2 3 4 5 / (213)	(214) 1 2 3 4 5 / (215)	(216) RIGHT 1 2 3 4 5 / (217) LEFT 1 2 3 4 5	(218) 1 2 3 4 5 / (219)	(220) 1 2 3 4 5 / (221)
7. Ankle	(222) 1☐R 3☐B 2☐L	(223) 1☐R 3☐B 2☐L	(224) 1☐R 3☐B 2☐L	(225) 1☐R 3☐B 2☐L		(226) 1☐R 3☐B 2☐L	(227) 1☐R 3☐B 2☐L
8. Feet	(228) 1☐R 3☐B 2☐L	(229) 1☐R 3☐B 2☐L	(230) 1☐R 3☐B 2☐L	(231) 1☐R 3☐B 2☐L		(232) 1☐R 3☐B 2☐L	(233) 1☐R 3☐B 2☐L

L BACK (234) 1 ☐ No findings — Skip to M
　　　　　　　　　　　　　　2 ☐ Findings — Continue with 1

1. Scoliosis . . . . 1.　(235) 1 ☐

2. Kyphosis . . . . 2.　(236) 1 ☐

3. Lordosis . . . . 3.　(237) 1 ☐

4. Tenderness

　　a. Sciatic notch . . . . . . 4a.　(238) 1 ☐ R　　2 ☐ L　　3 ☐ Both

　　b. Sacroiliac . . . . b.　(239) 1 ☐ R　　2 ☐ L　　3 ☐ Both

　　c. Other — Describe　　　☐ 240 1 ☐

　　_____

5. Limitation of motion

　　a. Cervical spine . . . . . . 5a.　(241) 1 ☐

　　b. Thoracic spine . . . . . . b.　(242) 1 ☐

　　c. Lumbar spine **flexion** . . c.　(243) 1 ☐

　　d. Lumbar spine, right
　　　　lateral flexion . . . . . d.　(244) 1 ☐

　　e. Lumbar spine, left
　　　　lateral flexion . . . . e.　(245) 1 ☐

　　f. Full extension . . . . . . f.　(246) 1 ☐

6. Pain on motion . . . . 6.　(247) 1 ☐ Negative　　　2 ☐ Positive

	Cervical	Thoracic	Low back	Diffuse	Uncertain
7. Flexion . . . . 7.	(248) 1 ☐	(249) 1 ☐	0 250 1 ☐	(251) 1 ☐	2 1 ☐
8. Extension . . . . 8.	(253) 1 ☐	(254) 1 ☐	(255) 1 ☐	(256) 1 ☐	1 ☐
9. Right lateral bending . . . 9.	(258) 1 ☐	(259) 1 ☐	(260) 1 ☐	(261) 1 ☐	(262) 1 ☐
10. Left lateral bending . . . . 10.	(263) 1 ☐	(264) 1 ☐	(265) 1 ☐	(266) 1 ☐	(267) 1 ☐
11. Right rotation. . . . . . . 11.	(268) 1 ☐	(269) 1 ☐	(270) 1 ☐	(271) 1 ☐	(272) 1 ☐
12. Left rotation . . . . 12.	(273) 1 ☐	(274) 1 ☐	0 275 1 ☐	(276) 1 ☐	(277) 1 ☐

M. STRAIGHT-LEG-RAISING TEST

　1. Right leg . . . . 1.　(278) 1 ☐ Neg.　2 ☐ Pos.

　2. Left leg . . . . 2.　(280) 1 ☐ Neg.　2 ☐ Pos.

　3. Increase —
　　a. On ankle (right leg) . . . 3a.　(279) ☐ Yes　2 ☐ No
　　b. Dorsiflexion (Left leg)　(281) ☐ ☼Ⅲ＋　2 ☐ No

N. OTHER SYSTEMS　(282) 1 ☐ No findings — Skip to 0
(Reticulo endcthelial, G.I., etc.)　　2 ☐ Findings — Describe ⟶

_____

_____

_____

_____

Sample Number
№ 98743

0. BLOOD PRESSURE

		TIME	SYSTOLIC	DIASTOLIC
1. Recumbent.	1.	⎯ ⎯ (283)	1 ☐ A.M. ○ 204 ⎯ ⎯ ⎯	○ 285 ⎯ ⎯ ⎯
2. Sitting	2.		2 ☐ P.M. ○ 207 ⎯ ⎯ ⎯	○ 288 ⎯ ⎯ ⎯

P. SUMMARY OF DIAGNOSTIC IMPRESSIONS

(289) 1 ☐ Normal; no abnormal findings
2 ☐ Abnormal significant finding noted **below**

		Severity Min.	Mod.	Sev.	Certainty (0–9)	ICD code
1. Cardiovascular						
a. _____ 1a.	(290)	1 ☐	2 ☐	3 ☐	○ 291 ⎯	○ 292 ⎯ ⎯ ⎯
b. _____ b.	(293)	1 ☐	2 ☐	3 ☐	○ 294 ⎯	○ 295 ⎯ ⎯ ⎯
c. _____ c.	(296)	1 ☐	2 ☐	3 ☐	○ 297 ⎯	○ 298 ⎯ ⎯ ⎯
2. Musculo-skeletal						
a. _____ 2a.	(299)	1 ☐	2 ☐	3 ☐	○ 300 ⎯	○ 301 ⎯ ⎯ ⎯
b. _____ b.	(302)	1 ☐	2 ☐	3 ☐	○ 303 ⎯	(304) ⎯ ⎯ ⎯
c. _____ c.	(305)	1 ☐	2 ☐	3 ☐	(306) 306 ⎯	(307) ⎯ ⎯ ⎯
3. Respiratory						
a. _____ 3a.	(308)	1 ☐	2 ☐	3 ☐	(309) ⎯	(310) ⎯ ⎯ ⎯
b. _____ b.	(311)	311 1 ☐	2 ☐	3 ☐	(312) 312	(313) ⎯ ⎯ ⎯
c. _____ c.	(314)	1 ☐	2 ☐	3 ☐	(315) ⎯	(316) ⎯ ⎯ ⎯
4. Other systems – Specify						
a. _____ 4a.	(317)	1 ☐	2 ☐	3 ☐	(318) ⎯	(319) ⎯ ⎯ ⎯
b. _____ b.	(320)	1 ☐	2 ☐	3 ☐	(321) 321	(322) ⎯ ⎯ ⎯
c. – _____ c.	(323)	1 ☐	2 ☐	3 ☐	(324) ⎯	○ 325 ⎯ ⎯ ⎯
5. _____						
a. _____ 5a.	1 (326)		2 ☐	3 ☐	(327) ⎯	(328) ⎯ ⎯ ⎯
b. _____ b.	(329)	1 ☐	2 ☐	3 ☐	(330) 330	(331) ⎯ ⎯ ⎯
c. _____ c.	(332)	1 ☐	2 ☐	3 ☐	(333) 333	(334) ⎯ ⎯ ⎯

Name of physician	Sample Number
	N⁰ 98743

87

L. Audiometry (Air)

HRA-12-10
FORMERLY HSM-425-10
(7-74)

Form Approved
O.M.B. No. 68-R1 I84

DEPARTMENT OF HEALTH, EDUCATION, AND WELFARE

PUBLIC HEALTH SERVICE
HEALTH RESOURCES ADMINISTRATION
NATIONAL CENTER FOR HEALTH STATISTICS

AUDIOMETRY (AIR)

HEALTH EXAMINATION SURVEY

a. Deck No.	b. Audio No.	c. Examiner No.
241	⓪01 _ _ _ _ _	⓪2 – –

▶ START *HERE IF SAMPLE NUMBER* EVEN

1. AIR CONDUCTION – RIGHT EAR

▶ *START HERE IF* SAMPLE *NUMBER ODD*

2. AIR CONDUCTION - LEFT EAR

Retest R with masking on L* (a)	Frequency (Hz) (b)	Hearing level (c)	Retest L with masking on R* (a)	Frequency (Hz) (b)	Hearing level (c)
⓪03	1000	⓪04	⓪31	1000	⓪32
⓪09	2000	⓪10	⓪37	2000	⓪38
⓪5	4000	⓪16	⓪43	4000	⓪44
⓪21	500	⓪22	⓪49	500	⓪50
⓪27	1000	⓪28	⓪55	1000	⓪56

3. CONDITION AFFECTING TEST RESULTS

Mark (X) only one

⓪59
1. ☐ None
2. ☐ Cold or sinusitis now
3. ☐ Ear discharge
4. ☐ Ringing or other noises in ears
5. ☐ Equipment defect**
6. ☐ Cold or sinusitis within one week
7. ☐ Earache within week
8. ☐ Other – *Describe* **

*Retest poorer ear with *A/C* masking on better ear only if differences in *A/C-HL* between the two ears is 40 *dB* or more

** Specify *frequencies* affected and describe 3

_____
_____
_____
_____
_____
_____

Comments

88

M. Respiratory Function Tests

HRA-12-9 (Formerly HSM-425-9)
4-74

DEPARTMENT OF HEALTH, EDUCATION, AND WELFARE

PUBLIC HEALTH SERVICE
HEALTH RESOURCES ADMINISTRATION
NATIONAL CENTER FOR HEALTH STATISTICS

HEALTH EXAMINATION SURVEY

RESPIRATORY FUNCTION TESTS

Form Approved
O.M.B. No. 68-R1 184

Deck No.

251

Room temperature

(000)1 __ __ ºC

A. SPIROMETER

1. Was test satisfactory? . . . . 1.

(002) 1 ☐ Yes   2 ☐ No — **Explain** 7

_____

_____

B. SINGLE BREATH DIFFUSING CAPACITY

1. inspired Co. 1.   1 0 0%

2. Small spirometer temperature . . . . 2.   (003) __ __ ºC

3a. Uncorrected barometric pressure . . . . . . 3a.   (004) __ __ __ . __ mm. Hg.

   b. Barometer temperature . . . . b.   (0)21 __ __ ºC

	TRIAL #1	TRIAL #2	TRIAL #3
4. inspired helium . . . . 4.	(005) __ __ . __ __	(010) __ __ . __ __	(015) __ __ . __ __
5. Expired helium percent . . . . 5.	(006) __ . __ __	(011) __ . __ __	(016) __ . __ __
6. Expired Co meter reading . . . . 6.	(007) __ __ . __	(012) __ __ . __	(017) __ __ . __
7. Breath holding time *cm . . . . 7.	(008) __ __ . __	(013) __ __ . __	(018) __ __ . __
8. Volume inspired V.C. (ATPS) ml . . . . 8.	(009) __ __ - __	(0)14 __ __ - __	(0)19 __ __ - __
9. Was test satisfactory? . . . . 9.	(020) 1 ☐ Yes 2 ☐ No — **Explain** →		

• From tracing — ½ inspiration point measured to onset of expiration

_____

NOTES

Sample Number

Nº 98743

89

HRA-12-24 /74)		Form Approved O.M.B. No. 68-W 184

DEPARTMENT OF HEALTH, EDUCATION, AND WELFARE
PUBLIC HEALTH SERVICE
HEALTH RESOURCES ADMINISTRATION
NATIONAL CENTER FOR HEALTH STATISTICS'

PHYSICIAN'S SUPPLEMENT
HEALTH EXAMINATION SURVEY

ASSURANCE OF CONFIDENTIALITY
All information which would permit identification of the individual will be held strictly confidential, will be used only by persons engaged in and for the purposes of the survey, and will not be disclosed or released to pthers for any other purposes (22 FR 1687).

Deck No. **082**

			Right	Left	Both	
1.	**Ocular fundi**					
	a. **Normal**	1a. (101)	1 ☐	2 ☐	3 ☐ →	If box 3 marked, **SKIP** to 2a
	b. **Fundus** not visualized	b. (102)	1 ☐	2 ☐	3 ☐	If box(es) 1, 2, or 3 marked, *SKIP* to 1m
	c. Globe absent	c. (103)	1 ☐	2 ☐	3 ☐ →	If box 3 marked, SKIP to 2a
	d. Increased light reflex	d. (104)	1 ☐	2 ☐	3 ☐	
	e. N&row orterioles	e. (105)	1 ☐	2 ☐	3 ☐	
	f. Tortuous arterioles	f. (106)	1 ☐	2 ☐	3 ☐	
	g. AV compression	g. (107)	1 ☐	2 ☐	3 ☐	
	h. Hemorrhage	h. (108)	1 ☐	2 ☐	3 ☐	
	i. Exudate	i. (109)	1 ☐	2 ☐	3 ☐	
	j. Venous engorgement	j. (110)	1 ☐	2 ☐	3 ☐	
	k. Popilledema	k. (111)	1 ☐	2 ☐	3 ☐	
	l. Disc **abnormal**	l. (112)	1 ☐	2 ☐	3 ☐	
	m. Lens opacities	m. (113)	1 ☐	2 ☐	3 ☐	
	n. Iritis	n. (114)	1 ☐	2 ☐	3 ☐	
	o. Othei – Specify 7	o. (115)	1 ☐	2 ☐	3 ☐	

2a.	Did a doctor ever tell you that you had protein, olbumin, blood or sugar in your urine?	2a. (116)	1 ☐ Yes – Ask b
			2 ☐ No – SKIP to 3

	b. Which?	b.	Yes	No
	Protein	(117)	1 ☐	2 ☐
	Albumin.	(118)	1 ☐	2 ☐
	Blood	(119)	1 ☐	2 ☐
	Sugar . . . . , ... , ...	(120)	1 ☐	2 ☐

3.	During the past 6 months have you had parasites or worms in your stools?	3. (121)	1 ☐ Yes
			2 ☐ No
			9 ☐ Don't know

SAMPLE NUMBER

N? 98743

4a. Do you have trouble with your bowels which makes you constipated or gives you diarrhea?	**4a.**	(122)	1 ☐ ⬚▯+ — constipated 2 ☐ Yes — diarrhea 3 ☐ No
b. How often do you usually have a bowel movement?	**b.**	(123)	1 ☐ Once a week or less often 2 ☐ 2-3 times a week 3 ☐ 4-6 times a week 4 ☐ Once a day s ☐ 2-3 times a day 6 ☐ 4 or more times a day
c. Have your movements ever been white, gray, dark black, or streaked with blood?	**c.**	(124)	1 ☐ ⬚▯+ — ▯&▯ d 2 ☐ No — SKIP to 5a

d. Which?

		Yes	No
White	(125)	1 ☐	2 ☐
Gray	(126)	1 ☐	2 ☐
Dark block	(127)	1 ☐	2 ☐
Streaked with blood	(128)	1 ☐	2 ☐

5a. Has a doctor ever told you that you had loss of blood from the stomach or bowels?	**5a.**	(129)	1 ☐ ⬚▯+ — ▯&▯ b 2 ☐ No — SKIP to 6a
b. Do you still have it?	**b.**	(130)	1 ☐ Yes 2 ☐ No s ☐ Don't know
c. How many years ago did you first have it?	**c.**	(131)	___ ___ Years ago
6a. Have you ever had an abdominal operation?	**6a.**	(132)	1 ☐ Yes — Ask b 2 ☐ No — SKIP to 7

b. Was it for . . .

		Yes	No
Tumor of the stomach, bowel, or colon?	(133)	1 ☐	2 ☐
Tumor or cyst of the womb or ovaries?	(134)	1 ☐	2 ☐

7. Do you have episodes (or "spells") of pain or discomfort in your abdomen or stomach of at least 3 days per month? (Don't count ones that go with a cold, sore throat, flu, or (for women) menstrual periods.)	**7.**	(135)	1 ☐ Yes 2 ☐ No

8. Do you have episodes (or "spells") of vomiting of at least 3 days per month? (Don't count ones that go with colds, sore throats, flu, or (for women) menstrual periods.)	**8.**	(136) 1 ☐ ⬚▯+ 2 ☐ No	**SAMPLE NUMBER** N? **98743**

9a. During the past year, have you had at least one drink of beer, wine, or liquor?	9a.	(137) 1 ☐ Yes – Ask b 2 ☐ No – *SKIP* to *Check* Item
b. How often do you drink?	b.	(138) 1 ☐ Every day 2 ☐ Just about every day 3 ☐ About 2 or 3 times a week 4 ☐ About 1–4 times a month 5 ☐ More than 3 but less than 12 times a year 6 ☐ No more than 2 or 3 times a year – *SKIP* to *Check* Item
c. Which do you most frequently drink -- beer, wine, or liquor?	c.	(139) 1 ☐ Beer 2 ☐ Wine 3 ☐ Liquor
d. When you drink (beer/wine/liquor), how much do you usually drink over 24 hours? (Enter an amount only for the one marked in *9c.*)	d.	(140) __ __Glasses of beer . .Glasses of wine __ __Drinks of liquor
CHECK ITEM		(141) 1 ☐ Female–Ask *10a* 2 ☐ Male – *END OF* QUESTIONNAIRE
10a. How old were you when your periods or menstrual cycles started?	10a.	(142) Years - Ask b 02 ☐ Haven't started yet – *END OF QUESTIONNAIRE*
b. Have they entirely stopped?	b .	(143) 1 ☐ Yes - Ask c ☐ ☐ – *SKIP* ☐ ☐
c. At what age?	c .	(144) __ -Years
11a. Have you taken birth control pills during the past 6 months?	1 la.	(145) 1 ☐ Yes – Ask b 2 ☐ No - SKIP to *12a*
b. Are you taking them now?	b.	(146) 1 ☐ Yes 2 ☐ No
12a. Are you or have you ever been pregnant?	12a.	(147) 1 ☐ Yes – Ask b 2 ☐ No – END Of QUESTIONNAIRE
b. What is the total number of pregnancies you have had?	b.	(148)__ -Number
c. What is the total number of miscarriages you have had?	c.	(149) __ -Number
d. What is the total number of live births you have had?	d.	(150) __ -Number
e. Are you pregnant now?	e.	(151) 1 ☐ Yes -Ask f 2 ☐ No 9 ☐ Don't know
f. Which month of pregnancy are you in?	f.	(152) __ -Month

SAMPLE NUMBER
Nº 98743

92

O. Report of Physical Findings

DEPARTMENT OF HEALTH, EDUCATION, AND WELFARE
PUBLIC HEALTH SERVICE
NATIONAL CENTER FOR HEALTH STATISTICS
ROCKVILLE, MD. 20852
HEALTH EXAMINATION SURVEY

REPORT OF PHYSICAL FINDINGS

Dear Doctor:

Recently the person named below **was a sample person who voluntarily participated as an examinee in the** Health Examination Survey conducted at special facilities of the U.S. Public Health Service. The objectives of the Survey are to obtain information on the health status of the U.S. population. The examination is not, and was not intended to be, a substitute for a visit to the examinee's physician, nor was it intended to be a complete examination. At the request of the examinee, however, we do send a report of certain selected procedures to his/her physician.

Reported below are physical findings which our physicians thought were significant and should be brought to your attention (i.e., for which no treatment had been sought and/or no history given). Also reported are some test reports and/or laboratory data. Although we are not engaged in follow-up or treatment of our findings, we appreciate the cooperation of our examinees and hope that we can contribute to their medical care by making this information available to you.

In addition to items listed below a separate letter will be sent reporting any significant conditions found on knee and hip X-rays if any are present.

Sincerely,

Arnold Engel

Arnold **Engel,** M.D.
Medical Advisor

Examinee's name and address ▶		Date of examination	Age	Height	Chest X-ray ☐ Encl. ☐ Not done	EKG ☐ Encl. ☐ Not done
			Sex	Weight		

MEDICAL	VISUAL ACUITY	BLOOD PRESSURE				
☐ N o **new significant findings**	R Eye L Eye	Systolic		Diastolic		
	20 / ___ 20 / ___					
	☐ Without glasses	**AUDIOGRAM – Decibels**				
	☐ With glasses	CPS	500	1000	2000	4000
	☐ With contacts	Right				
	☐ Not tested	Left				

		URINE	Neg	TR	1	2	3	4
Hematocrit _____ vol%		Albumin						
Hemoglobin _____ gm%		Sugar						
RBC count _____ mill/cc		Ph ☐5 ☐6 ☐7 ☐8 ☐9			SAMPLE NUMBER			
WBC count _____ thou/cc		Blood ☐ Pos c 1 Neg			№ 98743			

c 1 *SEE REVERSE SIDE FOR NOTES ON TESTS AND PROCEDURES*

93

NOTES ON TESTS AND PROCEDURES

Medical Examination – The physician's examination included the head and neck, chest (cardiopulmonary), abdomen, and extremities (musculoskeletal and neurological) - however, rectal, pelvic, and breast examinations were excluded.

X-Rays and EKG – A 12 lead EKG and A-P plus Lateral Chest X-rays were taken unless contraindicated. Knee and hip plus low back A-P X-rays were taken except on females age 49 or less. Copies enclosed are without interpretation – HES interpretations will be made later and used only as survey data.

Hematology – Screening limits *

Determination	Micro-hematocrit Vol. %	Cyanmet-hemoglobin Hgb Gm%	Coulter counter RBC/cc	Coulter counter WBC/cc
Adult Males	41 – 52	14.0 - 16.5	4.6 – 6.2 mill.	4.3 – 10 thou.
Adult Females	36 - 48	12.0 - 14.5	4.2 – 5.4 mill.	4.3 - 10 thou.
Pregnant Females	33 - 42	10.5 – 14.0	3.7 – 4.9 mill.	5.0 - 12 thou.

Urinalysis – Dip and read method using Ames Multistix.

Audiometry – Air conduction readings are reported in decibels with respect to audiometric zero (ISO - 1964), which is considered normal.

ROUGH GUIDELINES FOR dB REPORT AT 500 – 2000 cps.

25 dB or less – Hearing normal or more acute
30 – 40 dB – Near normal (difficulty with faint speech)
45 – 55 dB – Mild (difficulty with normal speech)
60 – 70 dB – Moderate (difficulty with loud speech)
75 – 100 dB – Severe (hears only amplified speech)
105 or more – Profound (usually cannot understand amplified speech)

Clinical Chemistry – Laboratory tests on blood are performed by a central laboratory. Results shown below, if any, are those received from the laboratory prior to the time this report was mailed. Additional results, if any, will be forwarded to you promptly when received.

BLOOD

Test	Result	Screening limits *	Test	Result	Screening limits *
Folate (s)	_____ mug%	5 – 30 mug%	T₄	_____	3.0 - 7.5 mcg%
Vitamin C (P)	_____ mg%	0.2 - 4.0 mg%	Murph –Pattee Test (if in&at ed)	_____	5.0 – 14.5 mcg%
Cholesterol	_____ mg%	260 or less	Total bilirubin (S)	_____ mg%	0.2 – 1.0 mg%
BUN	_____ mg%	30 mg% or less	SGOT (S)	_____ units	10 – 40 units
Creatinine	_____ mg%	1.50 mg% or less	Alk. phos. (S)	_____ I.U.	30 – 80 I.U. (SMA)
Sodium	_____ mEg/1	135 – 155	Uric acid (S) .	_____ mg%	2.5 - 7.0 mg%
Potassium	_____ mEg/1	3.5 – 5.0	Calcium (S)	_____ mg%	9.0 – 11.0 mg%
T 3 Euthy.	_____	0.88 – 1.10	Phosphrous (SorP)	_____ mg%	2.5 – 4.8 mg%
Hypo.	_____	Over – 1.10	(P) = Plasma (S) = Serum		
Hyper.	_____	Less – 0.88			

* Results outside the screening limits are considered to warrant further investigation of the examinee.

P. Vision Test

HRA-12-22
(8-23-74)

DEPARTMENT OF HEALTH, EDUCATION, AND WELFARE
PUBLIC HEALTH SERVICE
HEALTH RESOURCES ADMINISTRATION
NATIONAL CENTER FOR HEALTH STATISTICS

VISION TEST

HEALTH EXAMINATION SURVEY

ASSURANCE OF CONFIDENTIALITY — All information which would permit identification of the individual will be held strictly confidential, will only be used only by persons engaged in and for the purposes of the survey, and will not be disclosed or released to others for any other purposes (22 FR 1687).

a. Deck No. **163**

b. Name (Last, first, middle)

c. Age

d. Sex: 1 ☐ Male 2 ☐ Female

e. Sample No.

f. Examiner No. (Distance)

g. Name of Examiner (Distance)

h. Examiner No. (Near)

i. Name of Examiner (Near)

A. DISTANCE VISION

1. With or without correction
Mark (X) one

(099)
1 ☐ Wears glasses for test
2 ☐ Wears contact lenses for test
3 ☐ Forgot (glasses, contact lenses)
4 ☐ Does not wear either glasses or contact lenses

2. INSTRUCTION — Draw a diagonal line through each letter missed. Draw a horizontal line through sections of line not attempted and through top full line not attempted.

a. With correction — Both eyes (100)

Chart (a)	Line (b)	Number of errors allowed (c)	Score Mark (X) only one box (d)
Big L	400	0	00
K	200	0	01
K	160	0	02
DV	125	0	03
ZS	100	2	04
ORN / KH			
DV	80	0	05
HVC	60	1	06
ZHVD	50	1	07
OCVR	40	1	08
HOCRDS	30	2	09
KDVRZCOS	25	2	10
VRNHZDCSKO	20	3	11
ZSVDKHNORC	16	3	12

b. Without correction — Both eyes (101)

Chart (a)	Line (b)	Number of errors allowed (c)	Score Mark (X) only one box (d)
Big L	400	0	00
K	200	0	01
K	160	0	02
DV	125	0	03
ZS	100	2	04
ORN / KH			
DV	80	0	05
HVC	60	1	06
ZHVD	50	1	07
OCVR	40	1	08
HOCRDS	30	2	09
KDVRZCOS	25	2	10
VRNHZDCSKO	20	3	11
ZSVDKHNORC	16	3	12

c. With usual correction

(1) Left eye — (Odd numbers first) (102)

Chart (a)	Line (b)	Number of errors allowed (c)	Score Mark (X) only one box (d)
Big L	400	0	00
K	200	0	01
K	160	0	02
DV	125	0	03
ZS	100	2	04
ORN / KH			
DV	80	0	05
HVC	60	1	06
ZHVD	50	1	07
OCVR	40	1	08
HOCRDS	30	2	09
KDVRZCOS	25	2	10
VRNHZDCSKO	20	3	11
ZSVDKHNORC	16	3	12

(2) Right eye — (Even numbers first) (103)

Chart (a)	Line (b)	Number of errors allowed (c)	Score Mark (X) only one box (d)
Big L	400	0	00
K	200	0	01
K	160	0	02
DV	125	0	03
ZS	100	2	04
ORN / KH			
DV	80	0	05
HVC	60	1	06
ZHVD	50	1	07
OCVR	40	1	08
HOCRDS	30	2	09
KDVRZCOS	25	2	10
VRNHZDCSKO	20	3	11
ZSVDKHNORC	16	3	12

3. Test results: (104)
Mark (X) one
1 ☐ Test not done — Specify
2 ☐ Test unsatisfactory — Specify

1. With or without correction:

0_{105} 1 ☐ Wears glasses for test   3 ☐ Forgot (glasses, contact lenses)

     2 ☐ Wears contact lenses for test   4 ☐ Does not wear either glasses or contact lenses

2. Test using Sloan reading cards (both eyes) – Put horizontal line through words read correctly.

Selection (a)	Attempted (b)	Distance (cm) (c)	Smallest selection read satisfactorily Mark (X) one (d)	Number wrong (e)
500	0_{106} 1 ☐	0_{107} _ _ _	0 $_{108}$ 1 ☐	0_{109} _ _ _
350	(110) 1 ☐	0_{111} _ _ _	0 $_{112}$ 1 ☐	0_{113} _ _ _
250	0_{114} 1 ☐	0_{115} _ _ _	0 $_{116}$ 1 ☐	0_{117} _ _ _
200	0_{118} 1 ☐	0_{119} _ _ _	0 $_{120}$ 1 ☐	0_{121} _ _ _
150	0_{122} 1 ☐	0_{123} _ _ _	0_{124} r-1	0_{125} - - -
125	0_{126} 1 ☐	0_{127} - - - -	0 $_{128}$ 1 ☐	0_{129} _ _ _
100	0_{130} 1 ☐	0_{131} _ _ __	0 $_{132}$ 1 ☐	0_{133} - - - -
75	(134) 1 ☐	0_{135} _ _ _	0 $_{136}$ 1 ☐	0_{137} _ _ _
50	(138) $_{138}$ 1 ☐	0_{139} _ _ _	0_{140} 1 ☐	0_{141} _ _ _

3. Test using Keeney reading cards (both eyes) – Put horizontal line through word read correctly.

Selection (a)	Attempted (b)	Distance (cm) (c)	Smallest selection read satisfactorily Mark (X) one (d)	Number wrong (e)
130	0 $_{142}$ 1 ☐	0_{143} _ _ _	0_{144} 1 ☐	0_{145} _ _
120	0 $_{146}$ 1 ☐	0_{147} _ _ _	0_{148} 1 ☐	(149) _ _
85	0 $_{150}$ 1 ☐	0_{151} _ _ _	0_{152} ☐	0_{153} _ _
65	(154) $_{154}$ ☐	0_{155} _ _ _	0_{156} 1 ☐	0_{157} _ _
50	(158) $_{158}$ ☐	0_{159} _ _ _	0_{160} 1 ☐	0_{161} _ _
40	(162) $_{162}$ ☐	0_{163} _ _ _	0_{164} 1 ☐	0_{165} _ _
30	0_{166} 1 ☐	0_{167} _ _ _	0_{168} 1 ☐	0_{169} _ _
20	(170) $_{170}$ ☐	0_{171} _ _ _	(172) 1 ☐	0_{173} _ _

4. Conditions interfering with test:

0_{174} 1 ☐ Cannot read English   3 ☐ Difficulty speaking

     2 ☐ Cannot read   4 ☐ Other – Specify

C. NEAR VISION (FOR NON-ENGLISH OR ILLITERATES)

1. With or without correction:

(175) 1 ☐ Wears glasses for test   3 ☐ Forgot (glasses, contact lenses)

2 ☐ Wears contact lenses for test   4 ☐ Does not wear either glasses or contact lenses

▶ 2. Test using Sloan letters (both eyes)

Selection (a)	Distance (cm) (b)	Sloan letters — Draw a diagonal line through every letter missed. Draw a horizontal line through sections of line not attempted and through top full line not attempted. (c)								Errors allowed (d)	Score Mark (X) one (e)
500	(176) __ __ __	IT	IS	VY	HT	IN	TE	SN	TY	4	(177) 1 ☐
350	(178) __ __ __	CR	TE	TP	WH	CR	CS	AD	BN	4	(179) 179¹ ☐
250	(180) __ __ __	HE	YU	MD	TE	LR	YU	WE	TO	4	(181) 181¹ ☐
200	(182) __ __ __	OE	IN	LG	WE	AS	GT	TT	HE	4	(183) 1 ☐
150	(184) __ __ __	TE	WR	BU	FS	CR	TS	FR	TT	4	(185) 1 ☐
125	(186) __ __ __	TE	FS	AE	ED	TO	CE	FM	TE	4	(187) 1 ☐
100	(188) __ __ __	OE	DY	MY	NR	AD	ME	IF	HD	4	(189) 1 ☐
75	(190) __ __ __	VS	TO	FA	CS	GE	AE	ON	AD	4	(191) 191¹ ☐
50	(192) __ __ __	BW	TS	AE	OF	TO	KS	TE	TT	4	(193) 193¹ ☐

▶ 3. Test using Keeney letters (both eyes)

Selection (a)	Distance (cm) (b)	Keeney letters — Draw a diagonal line through every letter missed. Draw a horizontal line through sections of line not attempted and through top full line not attempted. (c)								Errors allowed (d)	Score Mark (X) one (e)
130	(194) __ __ __	WN	IN	TE	CE	GF	HN	ES	IT	4	(195) 1 ☐
120	(196) __ __ __	OE	PE	TO	DE	TE	PL	BS	WH	4	(197) 197¹ ☐
85	(198) __ __ __	WH	AR	AD	TO	AE	AG	TE	PS	'4	(199) 199¹ ☐
60	(200) __ __ __	WH	TE	LS	OF	NE	AD	OF	NS	4	(201) 1 ☐
so	(202) __ __ __	CS	WH	IL	TM	TO	TE	SN	WE	4	(203) 1 ☐
40	(204) __ __ __	RS	TT	AG	TE	AE	LE	LY	AD	4	(205) 1 ☐
30	(206) __ __ __	TT	WR	AY	FO	OF	GT	BS	DE	4	(207) 1 ☐
20	(208) __ __ __	ET	TR	SY	AD	HS	PE	ID	WL'	4	(209) 1 ☐

NAME _____   SAMPLE NUMBER _____

NEAR VISION TEST CARD

130   WHEN IN THE COURSE OF HUMAN EVENTS, IT BECOMES NECESSARY FOR

120   ONE PEOPLE TO DISSOLVE THE POLITICAL BANDS WHICH HAVE CONNECTED THEM

85   WITH ANOTHER, AND TO ASSUME AMONG THE POWERS OF THE EARTH, THE SEPARATE
AND EQUAL STATION TO

60   WHICH THE LAWS OF NATURE AND OF NATURE'S GOD ENTITLE THEM, A DECENT
RESPECT TO THE OPINIONS OF MANKIND REQUIRES THAT THEY SHOULD DECLARE THE

50   CAUSES WHICH IMPEL THEM TO THE SEPARATION. WE HOLD THESE TRUTHS TO BE
SELF-EVIDENT, THAT ALL MEN ARE CREATED EQUAL, THAT THEY ARE ENDOWED BY
THEIR CREATOR WITH CERTAIN UNALIENABLE

40   RIGHTS, THAT AMONG THESE ARE LIFE, LIBERTY, AND THE PURSUIT OF HAPPINESS.
THAT TO SECURE THESE RIGHTS, GOVERNMENTS ARE INSTITUTED AMONG MEN,
DERIVING THEIR JUST POWERS FROM THE CONSENT OF THE GOVERNED

30   THAT, WHENEVER ANY FORM OF GOVERNMENT BECOMES DESTRUCTIVE OF THESE ENDS,
IT IS THE RIGHT OF THE PEOPLE TO ALTER OR TO ABOLISH IT, AND TO
INSTITUTE NEW GOVERNMENT, LAYING ITS FOUNDATION ON SUCH PRINCIPLES AND
ORGANIZING ITS POWERS IN SUCH FORM, AS TO THEM SHALL SEEM MOST LIKELY TO

20   EFFECT THEIR SAFETY AND HAPPINESS. PRUDENCE INDEED, WILL DICTATE
THAT GOVERNMENTS LONG ESTABLISHED SHOULD NOT BE CHANGED FOR LIGHT AND
TRANSIENT CAUSES, AND ACCORDINGLY ALL EXPERIENCE HATH SHOWN, THAT
MANKIND ARE MORE DISPOSED TO SUFFER, WHILE EVILS ARE SUFFERABLE, THAN
TO RIGHT THEMSELVES BY ABOLISHING THE FORMS TO WHICH THEY ARE ACCUSTOMED.
BUT WHEN A LONG TRAIN OF ABUSES AND USURPATIONS

SLOAN NEAR VISION TEST CARD

500   IT IS VERY HOT IN THE SUN TODAY

350   COVER THE TOP WITH CRACKER CRUMBS AND BROWN IN A HOT OVEN.

250   HAVE YOU MAILED THE LETTER YOU WROTE TO YOUR NEPHEW? HE WILL
        EXPECT TO HEAR FROM YOU TOMORROW.

200   ONCE IN A LONG WHILE, AS A GREAT TREAT, HE TOOK ME DOWN TO HIS OFFICE.
        THIS COULD HAPPEN ONLY ON A SATURDAY MORNING WHEN THERE WAS NO SCHOOL.

150   THE WEATHER BUREAU FORECASTS COLDER TEMPERATURES FOR TONIGHT AND
        TOMORROW, WITH A WARMING TREND SETTING IN BY THURSDAY. LOW TEMPERATURES
        TONIGHT WILL BE IN THE LOW 30'S IN THIS AREA. TOMORROW'S HIGH WILL
        HIT ABOUT 37 DEGREES.

125   THE FUNDS ARE EXPECTED TO COME FROM THE SALE OF A TRACT OF LAND IN
        HERRING PARK. THE MONEY WILL NOT BECOME AVAILABLE UNTIL THE FIRST
        OF NEXT YEAR BUT OFFICIALS STATE THAT THEY CAN BEGIN ON SOME PARTS
        OF THE PROJECT AT ONCE.

100   ONE DAY MY NEIGHBOR ASKED ME IF I HAD MET THE WIDOW WHO HAD JUST MOVED
        INTO THE NEXT BLOCK. THAT NIGHT I HOBBLED DOWN THE STREET AND KNOCKED
        UPON HER DOOR. I EXPECTED TO FIND SOME SWEET, ALTHOUGH TOTTERING, LADY
        OF 80, BUT WHAT OPENED THE DOOR WAS THIS BLONDE. I PROPOSED TO HER
        IMMEDIATELY. SHE HAD A BETTER TELEVISION SET IN HER HOUSE THAN THE ONE
        I HAD IN MY COTTAGE.

75   VISITORS TO A FLORIDA CITRUS GROVE ARE OFTEN AMAZED TO SEE FULLY RIPE
        ORANGES BEING PICKED FROM A TREE WHICH IS ALSO FILLED WITH CLUSTERS OF
        FRAGRANT WHITE ORANGE BLOSSOMS--A GRAPHIC ILLUSTRATION OF THE TIME NATURE
        REQUIRES TO PRODUCE CITRUS FRUIT. UNLIKE MOST OTHER TYPES OF FRUIT, WHICH
        USUALLY NEED ONLY THREE TO FOUR MONTHS TO COMPLETE THEIR CYCLE FROM BLOSSOM
        TO MATURITY, CITRUS FRUITS REQUIRE TEN TO TWELVE MONTHS--AND THEY HAVE TO
        BE MONTHS OF SUNSHINE. THAT IS WHY A RELATIVELY SMALL SECTION, KNOWN AS
        THE "CITRUS BELT," WHICH EXTENDS ACROSS THE WAIST OF FLORIDA--AND WHERE
        THE SUN SHINES ALMOST EVERY DAY IN THE YEAR--PRODUCES NEARLY TWO-THIRDS
        OF ALL THE CITRUS FRUIT CONSUMED IN THE U.S.

50   BOW TIES ARE OF TWO KINDS, THOSE THAT ARE READY TIED AND THOSE THAT HAVE TO BE TIED. BOW TIES THAT HAVE TO BE TIED ARE PREFERRED, SINCE THE READY TIED ARE TOO PERFECT. IMPERFECTIONS IN THE TIE THAT HAS TO BE TIED SHOW THAT IT IS NOT MACHINE-MADE BUT HAND-WROUGHT. WHILE THE TIE THAT HAS TO BE TIED IS IMPERFECT IT SHOULD NOT BE TOO IMPERFECT. THAT IS TO SAY, ONE SIDE SHOULD NOT BE LONGER THAN THE OTHER SIDE, AND THE TIE SHOULD SIT HORIZONTALLY AND NOT AT AN ANGLE OF 45 DEGREES. TYING A BOW TIE DOES NOT COME NATURALLY.

Q. Speech Test (20-60 decibels)

DEPARTMENT OF HEALTH, EDUCATION, AND WELFARE
PUBLIC HEALTH SERVICE
HEALTH RESOURCES ADMINISTRATION
NATIONAL CENTER FOR HEALTH STATISTICS

SPEECH TEST
HEALTH EXAMINATION SURVEY

HRA-12-23A
(7-74)

a. Name (Last, first, middle)

b. Deck No. **242**

c. Sample No.   d. Segment No.   e. Serial No.   f. Column No.

i. Ear tested (103) 1 ☐ Right   2 ☐ Left

INSTRUCTIONS

Draw a horizontal line through all correct words. If after completing a list six or more words are missed, proceed to next list and increase decibel level by 10 until level 70 is reached. When 70 is reached go to Deck 243 (Blue paper)

g. List No. (101) **01**

h. Decibels — Mark (X) one (102) 1 ☐ 20   2 ☐ 30   3 ☐ 40   4 ☐ 50   5 ☐ 60

(104) X
1. WALKING'S MY FAVORITE EXERCISE.
(105)* 2. HERE'S a NICE QUIET PLACE to REST.
(106)* 3. OUR JANITOR SWEEPS the FLOORS EVERY NIGHT.
(107)* 4. it WOULD be MUCH EASIER IF EVERYONE would HELP.
(108)* 5. WE say GOOD MORNING and BEGIN to WORK.
(109)* 6. OPEN the WINDOW BEFORE you GO to BED.
(110)* 7. DO you THINK SHE SHOULD STAY HERE?
(111)* 8. HOW DO you FEEL about CHANGING?
(112)* 9. WHEN the TIME comes WE will GO.
(113)* 10. IT'S too LATE to MOVE OUT of the WAY.

RECORDER: Mark (X) only if this is the final level given.
(114) 1 ☐   Enter number of words missed →

j. List No. (115) **02**

k. Decibels — Mark (X) one (116) 1 ☐ 20   2 ☐ 30   3 ☐ 40   4 ☐ 50   5 ☐ 60

(118)* 1. the WATER'S TOO COLD for SWIMMING.
(119)* 2. WHY SHOULD I GET UP SO EARLY?
(120)* 3. SHINE YOUR own SHOES THIS TIME.
(121)* 4. IT'S RAINING right HERE in the ROOM.
(122)* 5. WHERE ARE you GOING this MORNING?
(123)* 6. YOU SHOULD COME HERE WHEN I CALL.
(124)* 7. DON'T TRY to GET OUT OF IT.
(125)* 8. WE LET LITTLE CHILDREN GO to the MOVIES.
(126)* 9. THERE ISN'T ENOUGH PAINT to FINISH.
(127)* 10. DO you WANT EGGS for BREAKFAST?

RECORDER: Mark (X) only if this is the final level given.
(128) 1 ☐   Enter number of words missed →

l. Ear tested (117) 1 ☐ Right   2 ☐ Left

101

List No. (129) 03

n. Decibels — Mark (X) one (130): 1 □ 20 2 □ 30 3 □ 40 4 □ 50 5 □ 60

o. Ear tested (131): 1 □ Right 2 □ Left

(132) 1. EVERYBODY should BRUSH TEETH BEFORE MEALS.
(133) 2. ONCE a YEAR EVERYTHING'S all RIGHT.
(134) 3. DON'T USE UP ALL the LETTER PAPER.
(135) 4. ANYTHING like THAT'S all RIGHT with me.
(136) 5. THOSE PEOPLE OUTSIDE OUGHT to SEE a DOCTOR.
(137) 6. the WINDOWS are SO DIRTY this MONTH I CAN'T see.
(138) 7. PLEASE PASS the BREAD and BUTTER FIRST.
(139) 8. DON'T FORGET to WRITE and PAY YOUR BILL.
(140) 9. DON'T LET the DOG OUT of the HOUSE.
(141) 10. THERE'S a GOOD BALLGAME this AFTERNOON.

RECORDER:
(142) Mark (X) only if this is the final level given.
Enter number of words missed →

p. List No. (143) 04

q. Decibels — Mark (X) one (144): 1 □ 20 2 □ 30 3 □ 40 4 □ 50 5 □ 60

r. Ear tested (145): 1 □ Right 2 □ Left

(146) 1. IF you WANT to GO IT'S all right.
(147) 2. THROW THESE OLD TIME MAGAZINES OUT.
(148) 3. DO you WANT to WASH UP in the STREAM?
(149) 4. it's a REAL DARK NIGHT SO WATCH your DRIVING.
(150) 5. I'LL CARRY YOUR PACKAGE for YOU.
(151) 6. DON'T YOU FORGET to SHUT OFF the WATER.
(152) 7. MOUNTAIN FISHING is my IDEA of a GOOD TIME.
(153) 8. FATHERS USED to SPEND more TIME with their CHILDREN.
(154) 9. BE CAREFUL NOT to BREAK the GLASSES.
(155) 10. I'M SORRIER THAN you for the mistake.

RECORDER:
(156) Mark (X) only if this is the final level given.
Enter number of words missed →

	x. Ear tested
	(173) 1 ☐ Right 2 ☐ Left

w. Decibels – Mark (X) one

(172) 1 ☐ 20 2 ☐ 30 3 ☐ 40 4 ☐ 50 5 ☐ 60

v. List No. (171)   06

(174) * 1. MUSIC ALWAYS MAKES me EER Up.

(175) * 2. my BROTHER'S in TOWN for a SHORT WHILE.

(176) * 3. WE - VE a FEW MILES off the MAIN ROAD.

(177) * 4. THIS SUIT NEEDS to GO to the CLEANERS.

(178) * 5. THEY ATE ENOUGH GREEN APPLES.

(179) * 6. have YOU BEEN SICK ALL THIS WEEK?

(180) * 7. WHERE HAVE YOU been WORKING LATELY?

(181) * 8. there's NOT ENOU TABLE ROOM in the KIT W?

(182) * 9. it's ARD to see WHERE W IS.

(183) * 10. LOOK OUT FOR NEW BUSINESS.

RECORDER:

(184) 1 ☐ *Mark (X) only if this is the ← final level given.*

Enter number of words missed ⟶

---

	u. Ear tested
	(159) 1 ☐ Right 2 ☐ Left

t. Decibels – Mark (X) one

(158) 1 ☐ 20 2 ☐ 30 3 ☐ 40 4 ☐ 50 5 ☐ 60

s. List No.   05

(157)

(160) . 1. YOU CAN CATCH the BUS ACROSS the STREET.

(161) * 2. TELL HER the NEWS on the PHONE.

(162) * 3. I'LL CATCH UP with YOU LATER.

(163) * 4. I'LL THINK it OVER AND CALL HER.

(164) * 5. I DON'T WANT to GO to the MOVIES.

(165) * 6. SEE a DENTIST IF YOUR TOOTH HURTS.

(166) * 7. PUT THAT COOKIE BACK in the BOX.

(167) * 8. you OUGHT to STOP FOOLING AROUND SO MUCH.

(168) * 9. TONIGHT THAT extra TIME'S Up.

(169)   10. HOW do you SPELL YOUR NAME?

RECORDER:

(170) 1 *Mark (X) only if this is the ← final level given.*

Enter number of words missed ⟶

List No. 07

(185) **07**

(186) **z. Decibels – Mark (X) one** 1□20 2□30 3□40 4□ 5□60

(187) **aa. Ear tested** 1□Right 2□Left

(188)* 1. I'll SEE YOU RIGHT AFTER LUNCH.

(189)* 2. I'll SEE YOU LATER this AFTERNOON.

(190)* 3. WHITE SHOES are AWFUL to KEEP CLEAN.

(191)* 4. YOU STAND OVER THERE UNTIL I MOVE.

(192)* 5. THERE'S a PIECE of CAKE LEFT for DINNER TONIGHT.

(193)* 6. DON'T WAIT for ME AT the FRONT CORNER.

(194)* 7. IT'S NO TROUBLE at ALL to TELL.

(195)* 8. HURRY UP with the MORNING PAPER.

(196)* 9. It DIDN'T SAY ANYTHING about a BIG RAIN.

(197)* 10. that DRUGSTORE PHONE CALL'S for YOU.

RECORDER: *Mark (X) only if this is the final level given.* (198) 1□

Enter number of words missed →

List No. 08

(199) **08**

(200) **cc. Decibels – Mark (X) one** 1□20 2□30 3□40 4□50 5□60

(201) **dd. Ear tested** 1□Right 2□Left

(202)* 1. BELIEVE ME it's TOO LATE.

(203)* 2. LET'S GET THAT CUP of COFFEE.

(204)* 3. LET'S get OUT of HERE BEFORE long.

(205)* 4. I HATE DRIVING IF IT'S at NIGHT.

(206)* 5. THERE WAS WATER in the CELLAR YESTERDAY.

(207)* 6. SHE'LL ONLY be GONE a FEW MINUTES.

(208)* 7. HOW do YOU KNOW WE'LL HAVE it SOON?

(209)* 8. CHILDREN LIKE CANDY AFTER HEAVY meals.

(210)* 9. NO GRASS grows when we DON'T GET RAIN.

(211)* 10. THEY'RE NOT LISTED in the NEW PHONE BOOK.

RECORDER: *Mark (X) only if this is the final level given.* (212) 1□

Enter number of words missed →

HRA-12-23A (7/74)

ee. List No. (213) **09**

ff. Decibels — Mark (X) one (214): 1□ 20 2□ 30 3□ 40 4□ 50 5□ 60

gg. Ear tested (215): 1□ Right 2□ Left

(216)* 1. WHERE CAN I FIND a PLACE to PARK?

(217)* 2. I LIKE THOSE BIG RED APPLES.

(218)* 3. YOU'LL get FAT by EATING CANDY.

(219)* 4. the COLOR SHOW'S OVER in the FALL.

(220)* 5. WHY DON'T they PAINT THEIR OTHER WALLS?

(221)* 6. HOW COME you ALWAYS GET to GO FIRST?

(222)* 7. WHAT ARE you HIDING UNDER your COAT?

(223)* 8. I SHOULD ALWAYS buy NEW cars.

(224)* 9. WHAT'S wrong with SUGAR and CREAM in my COFFEE?

(225)* 10. I'LL WAIT JUST ONE MINUTE.

RECORDER:

(226) 1□   Mark (X) only if this is the final level given.   Enter number of words missed →

---

hh. List No. (227) **10**

ii. Decibels — Mark (X) one (228): 1□ 20 2□ 30 3□ 40 4□ 50 5□ 60

ii. Ear tested (229): 1□ Right 2□ Left

(230)* 1. BUT we WON'T be READY to START.

(231)* 2. i DON'T KNOW what's WRONG WITH the CAR.

(232)* 3. it SURE TAKES a SHARP KNIFE to CUT MEAT.

(233)* 4. i HAVEN'T READ a NEW%% ER SINCE we got TELEVISION.

(234)* 5. the WEEDS ARE SPOILING THIS YARD.

(235)* 6. CALL ME a LITTLE LATER for BREAKFAST.

(236)* 7. DO you HAVE CHANGE for a FIVE-DOLLAR BILL?

(237)* 8. HOW ARE the things WE BOUGHT?

(238)* 9. i'd LIKE SOME ICE cream WITH MY PIE.

(239)* 10. i DON'T THINK I'LL HAVE DESSERT.

RECORDER:

(240) 1□   Mark (X) only if this is the final level given.   Enter number of words missed →

HRA-1223B
(7-74)

DEPARTMENT OF HEALTH, EDUCATION, AND WELFARE
PUBLIC HEALTH SERVICE
HEALTH RESOURCES ADMINISTRATION
NATIONAL CENTER FOR HEALTH STATISTICS

SPEECH TEST
HEALTH EXAMINATION SURVEY

b. Deck No. **243**

a. Name (Last, first, middle)

c. Sample No.   d. Segment No.   e. Serial No.   f. Column No.

INSTRUCTIONS

Draw a horizontal line through all correct words. If after completing a list six or more words are missed, proceed to next list and increase decibel level by 10 until level 80 is reached. After 80 is complete (END TEST).

(301) List No. **01**

(302) Decibels — Mark (X) one: 1 □ 70 2 □ 80

(303) Ear tested: 1 □ Right 2 □ Left

(304)* 1. WALKING'S MY FAVORITE EXERCISE.
(305)* 2. THERE'S A NICE QUIET PLACE TO REST.
(306)* 3. OUR JANITOR SWEEPS THE FLOORS EVERY NIGHT.
(307)* 4. IT WOULD BE MUCH EASIER IF EVERYONE would HELP.
(308) 5. WE say GOOD MORNING and BEGIN to WORK.
(309) 6. OPEN the WINDOW BEFORE you GO to BED.
(310)* 7. DO you THINK SHE SHOULD STAY HERE?
(311) 8. HOW DO you FEEL about CHANGING?
(312)* 9. WHEN the TIME comes, WE will GO.
(313) 10. IT'S too LATE to MOVE OUT of the WAY.

(314) RECORDER: Mark (X) only if this is the final level given. 1 □ | Enter number of words missed →

(315) List No. **02**

(316) Decibels — Mark (X) one: 1 □ 70 2 □ 80

(317) Ear tested: 1 □ Right 2 □ Left

(318)* 1. the WATER'S TOO COLD for SWIMMING.
(319)* 2. WHY SHOULD I GET up SO EARLY?
(320)* 3. SHINE YOUR own SHOES THIS TIME.
(321)* 4. IT'S RAINING right HERE in the ROOM.
(322)* 5. WHERE ARE you GOING this MORNING?
(323)* 6. YOU SHOULD COME HERE WHEN I CALL.
(324) 7. DON'T TRY to GET OUT OF IT.
(325)* 8. WE LET LITTLE CHILDREN GO to the MOVIES.
(326)* 9. THERE ISN'T ENOUGH PAINT to FINISH.
(327) 10. DO you WANT EGGS for BREAKFAST?

(328) RECORDER: Mark (X) only if this is the final level given. 1 □ | Enter number of words missed →

List No. 03

m. List No. (329) **03**

n. Decibels – Mark (X) one (330) 1☐ 70 2☐ 80

o. Ear tested (331) 1☐ Right 2☐ Left

(332)* 1. EVERYBODY should BRUSH TEETH BEFORE MEALS.

(333)* 2. ONCE a YEAR EVERYTHING'S all RIGHT.

(334)* 3. DON'T USE UP ALL the LETTE PAPER.

(335)* 4. ANYTHING like THAT'S all RIGH" with me.

(336)* 5. THOSE PEOPLE OUTSIDE OUGHT to SEE a DOCTOR.

(337)* 6. the WINDOWS are SO DIRTY this MONTH I CAN'T see.

(338)* 7. PLEASE PASS the BREAD and BITTER FIRST.

(339)* 8. DON'T FORGET to WRITE and RY YOUR BILL.

(340)* 9. DON'T LET the DOG OUT of th HOUSE.

(341)* 10. THERE'S a GOOD BALLGAME thi AFTERNOON.

RECORDER: (342) *Mark (X) only if this is the final level given.* 1☐ ← / Enter number of words missed →

List No. 04

p. List No. (343) **04**

q. Decibels – Mark (X) one (344) 1☐ 70 2☐ 80

r. Ear tested (345) 1☐ Right 2☐ Left

(346)* 1. IF you WANT to GO IT'S all right.

(347)* 2. THROW THESE OLD TIME MAGAZINES OUT.

(348)* 3. DO you WANT to WASH UP in the STREAM?

(349)* 4. it's a REAL DARK NIGHT SO WATCH your DRIVING.

(350)* 5. I'LL CARRY YOUR PACKAGE for YOU.

(351)* 6. DON'T YOU FORGET to SHUT OFF the WATER.

(352)* 7. MOUNTAIN FISHING is my IDEA of a GOOD TIME.

(353)* 8. FATHERS USED to SPEND more TIME with their CHILDREN.

(354)* 9. BE CAREFUL NOT to BREAK the GLASSES.

(355)* 10. I'M SORRIER THAN you for the mistake.

RECORDER: (356) *Mark (X) only if this is the final level given.* 1☐ ← / Enter number of words missed →

s. List No. (357) **05**

t. Decibels – Mark (X) one (358) 1 □ 70 2 □ 80

u. Ear tested (359) 1 □ Right 2 □ Left

(360)* 1. YOU CAN CATCH the BUS ACROSS the STREET.

(361)* 2. TELL HER the NEWS on the PHONE.

(362)* 3. I'LL CATCH UP with YOU LATER.

(363)* 4. I'LL THINK it OVER AND CALL HER.

(364)* 5. I DON'T WANT to GO to the MOVIES.

(365)* 6. SEE a DENTIST IF YOUR TOOTH HURTS.

(366)* 7. PUT THAT COOKIE BACK in the BOX.

(367)* 8. you OUGHT to STOP FOOLING AROUND so MUCH.

(368)* 9. TONIGHT THAT extra TIME'S UP.

(369)* 10. HOW do you SPELL YOUR NAME?

RECORDER:
(370) 1 □ *Mark (X) only if this is the final level given.*

Enter number of words missed →

---

v. List No. (371) **06**

w. Decibels – Mark (X) one (372) 1 □ 70 2 □ 80

x. Ear tested (373) 1 □ Right 2 □ Left

(374)* 1. MUSIC ALWAYS MAKES me CHEER UP.

(375)* 2. my BROTHER'S in TOWN for a SHORT WHILE.

(376)* 3. WE LIVE a FEW MILES off the MAIN ROAD.

(377)* 4. THIS SUIT NEEDS to GO to the CLEANERS.

(378)* 5. THEY ATE ENOUGH GREEN APPLES.

(379)* 6. have YOU BEEN SICK ALL THIS WEEK?

(380)* 7. WHERE HAVE YOU been WORKING LATELY?

(381)* 8. there's NOT ENOUGH TABLE ROOM in the KITCHEN.

(382)* 9. it's HARD to see WHERE HE IS.

(383)* 10. LOOK OUT FOR NEW BUSINESS.

RECORDER:
(384) 1 □ *Mark (X) only if this is the final level given.*

Enter number of words missed →

List No. 07

z. Decibels – Mark (X) one 386 1☐70 2☐80

aa. Ear tested 387 1☐Right 2☐Left

385 | 07

388* 1. I'll SEE YOU RIGHT AFTER LUNCH.

389* 2. I'll SEE YOU LATER this AFTERNOON.

390* 3. WHITE SHOES are AWFUL to KEEP CLEAN.

391* 4. YOU STAND OVER THERE UNTIL I MOVE.

392* 5. THERE'S a PIECE of CAKE LEFT for DINNER TONIGHT.

393* 6. DON'T WAIT for ME AT the FRONT CORNER.

394* 7. IT'S NO TROUBLE at ALL to TELL.

395* 8. HURRY UP with the MORNING PAPER.

396* 9. it DIDN'T SAY ANYTHING about a BIG RAIN.

397* 10. that DRUGSTORE PHONE CALL'S for YOU.

RECORDER:
Enter number of words missed →
398 1☐ Mark (X) only if this is the ←final level given.

List No. 08

cc. Decibels – Mark (X) one 400 1☐70 2☐80

dd. Ear tested 401 1☐Right 2☐Left

399 | 08

402* 1. BELIEVE ME it's TOO LATE.

403* 2. LET'S GET THAT CUP of COFFEE.

404* 3. LET'S get OUT of HERE BEFORE long.

405* 4. I HATE DRIVING IF IT'S at NIGHT.

406* 5. THERE WAS WATER in the CELLAR YESTERDAY.

407* 6. SHE'LL ONLY be GONE a FEW MINUTES.

408* 7. HOW do YOU KNOW WE'LL HAVE it SOON?

409* 8. CHILDREN LIKE CANDY AFTER HEAVY meals.

410* 9. NO GRASS grows when we DON'T GET RAIN.

411* 10. THEY'RE NOT LISTED in the NEW PHONE BOOK.

RECORDER:
Enter number of words missed →
412 1☐ Mark (X) only if this is the ←final level given.

List No. 09

ee. List No. **09**

ff. Decibels — Mark (X) one (414): 1 □ 70   2 □ 80

gg. Ear tested (415): 1 □ Right   2 □ Left

(416)* 1. WHERE CAN I FIND a PLACE to PARK?

(417)* 2. I LIKE THOSE BIG RED APPLES.

(418) 3. YOU'LL get FAT by EATING CANDY.

(419)* 4. the COLOR SHOW'S OVER in the FALL.

(420)* 5. WHY DON'T they PAINT THEIR OTHER WALLS?

(421)* 6. HOW COME you ALWAYS GET to GO FIRST?

(422)* 7. WHAT ARE you HIDING UNDER your COAT?

(423)* 8. I SHOULD ALWAYS buy NEW cars.

(424)* 9. WHAT'S wrong with SUGAR and CREAM in my COFFEE?

(425)* 10. I'LL WAIT JUST ONE MINUTE.

RECORDER:

(426) 1 □ ← final level given.   Mark (X) only if this is the final level given.

Enter number of words missed ⟶

List No. 10

hh. List No. **10** (427)

ii. Decibels — Mark (X) one (428): 1 □ 70   2 □ 80

jj. Ear tested (429): 1 □ Right   2 □ Left

(430)* 1. BUT we WON'T be READY to START.

(431)* 2. I DON'T KNOW what's WRONG WITH the CAR.

(432)* 3. it SURE TAKES a SHARP KNIFE to CUT MEAT.

(433) 4. I HAVEN'T READ a NEWSPAPER SINCE we got TELEVISION.

(434) 5. the WEEDS ARE SPOILING THIS YARD.

(435)* 6. CALL ME a LITTLE LATER for BREAKFAST.

(436)* 7. DO you HAVE CHANGE for a FIVE OR a BILL?

(437) 8. HOW ARE the things WE BOUGHT?

(438)* 9. I'd LIKE SOME ICE cream WITH MY PIE.

(439) 10. I DON'T THINK I'LL HAVE DESSERT.

RECORDER:

(440) 1 □ ← final level given.   Mark (X) only if this is the final level given.

Enter number of words missed ⟶

☆ U.S. GOVERNMENT PRINTING OFFICE : 1978 260-937/15

VITAL AND HEALTH STATISTICS PUBLICATIONS SERIES

Formerly Public Health Service Publication No. 1000

Series 1. Programs and Collection Procedures.-Reports which describe the general programs of the National Center for Health Statistics and its offices and divisions, data collection methods used, definitions, and other material necessary for understanding the data.

Series 2. Data Evaluation and Methods Research. -Studies of new statistical methodology including experimental tests of new survey methods, studies of vital statistics collection methods, new analytical techniques, objective evaluations of reliability of collected data, contributions to statistical theory.

Series 3. Analytical Studies. -Reports presenting analytical or interpretive studies based on vital and health statistics, carrying the analysis further than the expository types of reports in the other series.

Series 4. Documents and Committee Reports. -Final reports of major committees concerned with vital and health statistics, and documents such as recommended model vital registration laws and revised birth and death certificates.

Series 10. Data from the Health Interview Survey. —Statistics on illness; accidental injuries; disability; use of hospital, medical, dental, and other services; and other health-related topics, based on data collected in a continuing national household interview survey.

Series 11. Data from the Health Examination Survey.—Data from direct examination, testing, and measurement of national samples of the civilian, noninstitutionalized population provide the basis for two types of reports: (1) estimates of the medically defined prevalence of specific diseases in the United States and the distributions of the population with respect to physical, physiological, and psychological characteristics; and (2) analysis of" relationships among the various measurements without reference to an explicit finite universe of persons.

Series 12. Data from the Institutionalized Population Surveys. -Discontinued effective 1975. Future reports from these surveys will be in Series 13.

Series 13. Data on Health Resources Utilization.-Statistics on the utilization of health manpower and facilities providing long-term care, ambulatory care, hospital care, and family planning services.

Series 14. Data on Health Resources: Manpower and Facilities. -Statistics on the numbers, geographic distribution, and characteristics of health resources including physicians, dentists, nurses, other health occupations, hospitals, nursing homes, and outpatient facilities.

Series 20. Data on Mortality.-Various statistics on mortality other than as included in regular annual or monthly reports. Special analyses by cause of death, age, and other demographic variables; geographic and time series analyses; and statistics on characteristics of deaths not available from the vital records, based on sample surveys of those records.

Series 21. Data on Natality, Marriage, and Divorce. -Various statistics on natality, marriage, and divorce other than as included in regular annual or monthly reports. Special analyses by demographic variables; geographic and time series analyses; studies of fertility; and statistics on characteristics of births not available from the vital records, based on sample surveys of those records.

Series 22. Data from the National Mortality and Natality Surveys. -Discontinued effective 1975. Future reports from these sample surveys based on vital records will be included in Series 20 and 21, respectively.

Series 23. Data from the National Survey of Family Growth. -Statistics on fertility, family formation and dissolution, family planning, and related maternal and infant health topics derived from a biennial survey of a nationwide probability sample of ever-married women 1544 years of age.

For a list of titles of reports published in these series, write to: Scientific and Technical Information Branch
National Center for Health Statistics
Public Health Service
Hyattsville, Md. 20 782